**CHIRON VACCINES
AT YOUR SERVICE**

Lyme Borreliosis and Tick-Borne Encephalitis

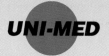

UNI-MED Verlag AG

CIP-Titelaufnahme der Deutschen Bibliothek
Oschmann, Patrick:
Lyme Borreliosis and Tick-Borne Encephalitis/Patrick Oschmann, Peter Kraiczy, John Halperin und Volker Brade (Hrsg.).-
1. Auflage - Bremen: UNI-MED, 1999
ISBN 3-89599-449-9

© 1999   by UNI-MED Verlag AG, Kurfürstenallee 130, D-28211 Bremen, Germany
International Medical Publishers

Printed in Germany

This work is subject to copyright. All rights are reserved, whether the whole or part of the material is concerned, specifically the rights of translation, reprinting, reuse of illustrations, recitation, broadcasting, reproduction on microfilm or in any other way and storage in data banks. Violations are liable for prosecution under the German Copyright Law.

The use of general descriptive names, registered names, trademarks, etc. in this publication does not imply, even in the absence of a specific statement, that such names are exempt from the relevant protective laws and regulations and therefore free for general use.

Product liability: The publishers cannot guarantee the accuracy of any information about the application of operative techniques and medications contained in this book. In every individual case the user must check such information by consulting the relevant literature.

MEDICINE - STATE OF THE ART

UNI-MED Verlag AG, one of the leading medical publishing companies in Germany, presents its highly successful series of scientific textbooks, covering all medical subjects. The authors are specialists in their fields and present the topics precisely, comprehensively, and with the facility of quick reference in mind. The books will be most useful for all doctors who wish to keep up to date with the latest developments in medicine.

Foreword to the first English edition

Although only six months have passed since the first German edition of this book appeared, its success in German-speaking countries and the worldwide distribution of the clinical picture have already persuaded the authors to prepare an English version. The clinical picture of Lyme borreliosis differs in certain aspects in Europe and the United States. For this reason we were very pleased that one of the most widely acknowledged experts from the United States, Prof. Halperin, immediately agreed to join our team of authors. The swift publication of the English edition would not have been possible without the generous support of the publisher and Chiron Behring, Marburg, Germany.

Giessen, Frankfurt, Manhasset, June 1999
P. Oschmann
P. Kraiczy
J. Halperin
V. Brade

Foreword and acknowledgements

Lyme borreliosis and spring-summer encephalitis are the most common tick-borne diseases in the western hemisphere. Despite this, there is often still a lack of clarity about the delimitation of the two entities in relation to their epidemiological significance, clinical picture, diagnostic methods, and prophylactic measures, particularly protective inoculation. In the past this has led to misunderstandings and imprecise medical procedures.

This book has been written as a compact introduction for physicians in all specialties in hospital and general practice. It is intended to provide practice-oriented information, but at the same time to describe the theoretical background in as much detail as is required to understand the pathogenetic relationships. Those who require more detailed information can make use of the literature references at the end of each chapter. In all the descriptions, value was placed on clarity and rapid availability of information, so scientific references were deliberately omitted.

The authors are members of an interdisciplinary expert group of microbiologists and physicians who have been working in the area of tick-borne diseases for many years. The personal experience of each of the authors, accumulated through daily work with patients in special clinics or by confrontation with complicated questions in laboratory diagnosis, thus forms one important pillar of this book. The authors have also gathered scientific understanding of this disease through publications, symposia, and involvement in multicenter studies. The idea of writing this book came from the last Frankfurt-Giessen Borrelia symposium held in Frankfurt in May 1997.

Completion of the book in the short time it has taken was possible only through the close cooperation of many colleagues, mostly employees of Giessen and Frankfurt University Hospitals. In this connection we would like to offer particular thanks to our secretaries Frau Hardt and Frau Glaser for their excellent work preparing the manuscript. We thank the publishers for smooth and straightforward collaboration. Our special thanks are due to Prof. Brade, director of the Institute of Medical Microbiology at Frankfurt University Hospital and Prof. Dorndorf, head of Giessen University Neurology Clinic for much encouragement and general support and for authorship. Finally, but not least, we would like to thank our wives Claudia and Andrea for their constant understanding when we had to dedicate our evenings and weekends to the book.

We hope that the book fulfills the requirements of the readers, and are always grateful for constructive criticism from practicing physicians.

Giessen and Frankfurt, August 1998

P. Oschmann
P. Kraiczy

Preface

The tick-borne diseases now known as Lyme borreliosis have been intensively studied since the discovery of their etiology. The natural history and clinical course of this unusually varied human infection and the complex environmental relationships involving the pathogen present a fascinating picture which has come to light in just fifteen years or so.

The diagnosis of the disease, which develops in stages and tends to relapse and become chronic, can pose a variety of problems for the practicing physician. Only some of its many organ manifestations correspond to a clinical entity which can be easily recognized. Others only produce a picture of limited specificity or even completely uncharacteristic symptoms.

The diagnostic difficulties can be made worse by the limited informative value of specific laboratory findings. Inconsequential residual titers or clinically inapparent infections, courses which remain or become seronegative, the absence of a consistently valid serological activity indicator, and the different antigen spectra of different species and strains of Borrelia can make unambiguous laboratory diagnosis more difficult and require the results to be viewed in the light of the clinical situation. The decision is always that of the practicing physician. To make it, he must be well acquainted with the diverse clinical pictures and the difficulties of etiological laboratory diagnosis.

TBE, which is transmitted by the same vector but is caused by a virus, is characterized by an easily recognized clinical picture. Its serological diagnosis is reliable and can indicate the activity of the infection. In Germany it occurs much less often than Lyme borreliosis and is limited to certain endemic areas in the south of the country. Information about these areas, gathered laboriously in the last 40 years, forms the basis of the prophylactic measures which are so important, in particular providing the indication for the well-established active protective inoculation.

Detailed information about the two native tick-borne, but otherwise fundamentally different, diseases is now essential in everyday clinical practice. This book provides an excellent introduction to the subject.

Cologne, May 1998 *Prof. Dr. R. Ackermann*

Authors

Prof. Dr. rer. nat. habil. Georg Acker
Department of Biological Electron Microscopy
Bayreuth University
Universitätsstrasse 30
D-95440 Bayreuth
Chapter 2.1.

Prof. Dr. med. Volker Brade
Institute of Medical Microbiology
Frankfurt University Hospital
Paul-Ehrlich-Strasse 40
D-60596 Frankfurt
Chapters 2., 4., 6.1.3., 6.2.3.

Dr. med. Michael Hahn
Department of Neurology
University of Giessen
Am Steg 14
D-35385 Giessen
Chapter 3.

Dr. John Halperin, MD
Department of Neurology
North Shore University Hospital
Manhasset, NY 11030, USA
Chapter 9.

Dr. med. Klaus-Peter Hunfeld
Institute of Medical Microbiology
Frankfurt University Hospital
Paul-Ehrlich-Strasse 40
D-60596 Frankfurt
Chapters 6.1.3., 6.2.3.

Priv.-Doz. Dr. Reinhard Kaiser
Department of Neurology
University of Freiburg
Breisacher Strasse 64
D-79106 Freiburg
Chapters 5.2., 6.2.1.-2., 7.2., 8.3.

Dr. phil. nat. Peter Kraiczy
Institute of Medical Microbiology
Frankfurt University Hospital
Paul-Ehrlich-Strasse 40
D-60596 Frankfurt
Chapter 2.4.

Dr. med. Patrick Oschmann
Department of Neurology
University of Giessen
Am Steg 14
D-35385 Giessen
Chapters 1.3., 5.1., 6.1.1.-2., 7.1., 8.1.-2.

Claudia Schäfer
Department of Neurology
University of Giessen
Am Steg 14
D-35385 Giessen
Chapter 3.

Dr. med. Jörg Schulze
Institute of Medical Microbiology
Frankfurt University Hospital
Paul-Ehrlich-Strasse 40
D-60596 Frankfurt
Chapters 6.1.3., 6.2.3.

Contents

1. Introduction (P. Oschmann) 16

2. Characteristics of the pathogen (P. Kraiczy, G. Acker, V. Brade) 20
  2.1. Lyme borreliosis 20
   2.1.1. Taxonomic classification 20
   2.1.2. Morphology 21
   2.1.3. Culture conditions 22
   2.1.4. Molecular biology aspects 22
   2.1.5. Antigen structure and antigenic diversity of *B. burgdorferi* s.l. 24
  2.2. Tick-borne encephalitis (TBE) 25
   2.2.1. Taxonomic classification and structure of the TBE virus 25
   2.2.2. Molecular biology aspects 26
   2.2.3. Antigen structure of the TBE virus 26

3. Tick ecology and epidemiology (C. Schäfer, M. Hahn, P. Oschmann) 30
  3.1. Tick ecology 30
   3.1.1. Ticks — a general introduction 30
   3.1.2. Ixodes ricinus 30
  3.2. Epidemiology 32
   3.2.1. Lyme borreliosis 32
   3.2.2. Tick-borne encephalitis (TBE) 34

4. Pathogenesis and immune defense (V. Brade, P. Kraiczy) 42
  4.1. Lyme borreliosis 42
   4.1.1. Pathogenesis 42
    4.1.1.1. Local infection 42
    4.1.1.2. Dissemination 43
    4.1.1.3. Acute organ manifestations 44
    4.1.1.4. Chronic organ manifestations 44
   4.1.2. Immune defense 45
    4.1.2.1. Preimmune phase 45
    4.1.2.2. Immune phase 45
     4.1.2.2.1. Reinfections 45
     4.1.2.2.2. Persistence of *Borreliae* 46
    4.1.2.3. Immunopathology 46
  4.2. Tick-borne encephalitis (TBE) 47
   4.2.1. Pathogenesis 47
   4.2.2. Immune defense 47

5. Clinical symptoms (P. Oschmann, R. Kaiser) 52
  5.1. Lyme borreliosis 52
   5.1.1. Course of infection and stages 52
   5.1.2. Organ manifestations and the associated syndromes 53
    5.1.2.1. Dermatoborreliosis 54
     5.1.2.1.1. Erythema (chronicum) migrans (E[C]M) — stage I 54
     5.1.2.1.2. Lymphadenosis cutis benigna (LCB) — stage I/III 55
     5.1.2.1.3. Acrodermatitis chronica atrophicans (ACA) — stage III 56

                5.1.2.1.4. Circumscribed scleroderma, lichen sclerosis et atrophicus (stage III) 57
        5.1.2.2. Neuroborreliosis..57
                5.1.2.2.1. Meningoradicul(oneur)itis (stage II, Garin-Bujadoux-Bannwarth syndrome)......................59
                5.1.2.2.2. Meningomyel(oradicul)itis (stage II) 61
                5.1.2.2.3. Meningitis (stage II) 61
                5.1.2.2.4. Meningoencephal(oradicul)itis (stage II) 62
                5.1.2.2.5. Cerebrovascular neuroborreliosis (stage II/III) 63
                5.1.2.2.6. Progressive encephalomyelitis (stage III)...65
                5.1.2.2.7. Lyme encephalopathy 66
                5.1.2.2.8. Acute and chronic neuritis, myositis, and fasciitis (stage II/III) 66
        5.1.2.3. Internistic manifestations 68
                5.1.2.3.1. Lyme arthritis 68
                5.1.2.3.2. Lyme carditis 69
        5.1.2.4. Ophthalmoborreliosis 69
5.2. Tick-borne encephalitis...70
    5.2.1. Course of the disease 70
        5.2.1.1. Prodromal phase 71
        5.2.1.2. Manifestation phase..72
    5.2.2. Organ manifestations and syndromes 72
        5.2.2.1. Meningitis...72
        5.2.2.2. Encephalitis 73
        5.2.2.3. Encephalomyelitis and radiculitis 74
        5.2.2.4. Manifestations outside the nervous system 75

6. Diagnostics (K.-P. Hunfeld, P. Oschmann, R. Kaiser, J. Schulze, V. Brade) 80

6.1. Lyme borreliosis 80
    6.1.1. Cardinal symptoms and instrumental examinations..80
    6.1.2. Nonspecific laboratory changes in blood, CSF, and synovial fluid..82
    6.1.3. Microbiological diagnosis of Lyme borreliosis 84
        6.1.3.1. Diagnostic methods for direct pathogen detection in Lyme borreliosis....................................86
                6.1.3.1.1. Direct microscopic detection 86
                6.1.3.1.2. Detection of the pathogen by culture..86
                6.1.3.1.3. Antibiotic sensitivity testing of *Borrelia burgdorferi* s.l. 87
                6.1.3.1.4. Direct detection with the aid of the polymerase chain reaction 88
                6.1.3.1.5. Detection of Borrelia-specific antigens in clinical specimens 90
                6.1.3.1.6. Methods of differentiating species..90
        6.1.3.2. Indirect detection of the pathogen (serological detection of antibodies)..................................91
                6.1.3.2.1. Stage-dependent antibody kinetics in Lyme borreliosis 91
                6.1.3.2.2. Serological tests in Lyme borreliosis diagnostics 92
        6.1.3.3. Rational standard serological diagnostics and interpretation of findings in Lyme borreliosis ...96
                6.1.3.3.1. Special problems in the interpretation of positive borreliosis serology findings 99
        6.1.3.4. Detection of specific antibody synthesis in the cerebrospinal fluid in neuroborreliosis............99
        6.1.3.5. Possible sources of error in serological Lyme borreliosis diagnostics...................................102
        6.1.3.6. Need for further standardization of tests..102
        6.1.3.7. Summary and critical assessment 103
6.2. Tick-borne encephalitis (TBE) 103
    6.2.1. Principal symptoms and instrumental examinations 103
    6.2.2. Nonspecific laboratory changes in blood and cerebrospinal fluid 104
    6.2.3. Microbiological diagnostics 105
        6.2.3.1. Direct microbiological methods (detection of the virus) 105
                6.2.3.1.1. Culture of the virus and electron microscopy 105
                6.2.3.1.2. Direct detection of TBE virus by RT-PCR 106

    6.2.3.2. Indirect detection methods (detection of antibodies) 106
        6.2.3.2.1. ELISA 106
        6.2.3.2.2. Antibody kinetics and interpretation of findings in the course of an TBE infection 107
        6.2.3.2.3. Detection of antibodies in the cerebrospinal fluid in TBE 107
    6.2.3.3. Critical assessment 108

7. Therapy and prognosis (P. Oschmann, R. Kaiser) 112
7.1. Lyme borreliosis 112
    7.1.1. Therapy 112
        7.1.1.1. Therapeutic principles 112
        7.1.1.2. Pragmatic therapy 113
            7.1.1.2.1. Therapy of stage I 113
            7.1.1.2.2. Therapy of stage II 114
            7.1.1.2.3. Therapy of stage III 114
            7.1.1.2.4. Therapy during pregnancy 115
            7.1.1.2.5. Assessment of the therapeutic outcome 115
    7.1.2. Prognosis, relapse, treatment resistance, and delayed cure 117
7.2. Tick-borne encephalitis (TBE) 118
    7.2.1. Therapy 118
    7.2.2. Prognosis 119

8. Prophylactic measures (P. Oschmann, R. Kaiser) 124
8.1. General protection measures 124
    8.1.1. General protection against ticks 124
    8.1.2. Removal of ticks 124
    8.1.3. Tick control 125
8.2. Lyme borreliosis 125
8.3. Tick-borne encephalitis 127

9. Special aspects of Lyme borreliosis and tick-borne encephalitis in the United States (J. Halperin) 132
9.1. Introduction 132
9.2. Characteristics of the pathogen 132
9.3. Tick ecology and epidemiology 133
9.4. Pathogenesis 133
9.5. Clinical Symptoms 133
9.6. Diagnostics 135
9.7. Therapy and Prognosis 136
9.8. Prophylactic measures 136

10. List of abbreviations 139

Index 141

Introduction

1. Introduction

The existence of tick-borne pathogens has been known since the beginning of the century. In 1909 *Rickett* discovered the eponymous genus of bacteria responsible for Rocky Mountain spotted fever — Rickettsia. The 1930s saw the first reports of **tick-borne encephalitis encephalitis (TBE)**, from the far-eastern part of Russia; the organism which causes the disease, a flavivirus, was isolated in 1937. In 1931 *Schneider* described a similar clinical picture in Austria, calling it 'epidemic acute serous meningitis', which is why, in older literature TBE is also referred to as Schneider's disease. The disease did not enter the Central European consciousness until after the Second World War. The basic virological, serological, and epidemiological details were established mainly in the 1950s and 1960s. TBE is now the most important arboviral disease and endemic viral encephalitis in Central and Eastern Europe (☞ Section 3.2). The viruses are not uniformly distributed across these countries, but are confined, unlike *B. burgdorferi*, to areas of endemic occurrence.

> TBE occurs mainly in the southern and eastern parts of Germany, in Austria, the Czech and Slovak Republics, the Balkans, and the states which were formerly part of the USSR.

The terms

- Tick-borne encephalitis (TBE)
- Central European encephalitis (CEE)
- Russian spring-summer encephalitis (RTBE) and
- Spring-summer encephalitis (TBE)

are often used as synonyms, even though, as Sections 2.2 and 3.2.2 make clear, this is not quite correct.

The history of the discovery of **Lyme borreliosis** has two stages. In 1909 the Swedish dermatologist *Artvid Afzelius* gave a report at a meeting of the Stockholm Dermatological Society, in which he described the case of an elderly woman suffering from **erythema migrans** which was probably caused by *Ixodes reduvii* (syn. *Ixodes ricinus*). Long before this, in 1883, *Buchwald* had described a condition called **acrodermatitis chronica atrophicans** and subsequently, in 1943, *Bäfverstedt* described a disease known as **lymphocytoma cutis** or **lymphadenosis cutis benigna**. In the decades that followed, European scientists succeeded in demonstrating the infectious nature of these dermatoses on the basis of numerous tick-bite case histories and human-to-human transmission studies, and in making successful treatment a likely prospect with penicillin. For the time being, however, definitive isolation of the pathogen was to elude them, despite *Lehnhof*'s article of 1947 concerning the detection of spirochetes in skin biopsy material from patients with erythema migrans. There had already been reports of rheumatic and radicular-neuritic concomitant symptoms in isolated cases of acrodermatitis chronica atrophicans. *Garin* and *Bujadoux* (1922) were the first to describe a clinical picture characterized by meningitis with accompanying radicular deficits, which occurred after a tick bite, coining the term "paralysie par les tiques". Detailed descriptions followed — from *Bannwarth* in 1941 and, 20 years later, from *Schaltenbrand*. The latter author drew attention to the acute and chronic multisystemic character of this disease in numerous case series and gave a detailed account of the attack on the nervous system, describing it as meningoencephaloradiculomyelitis. Although he suspected that it was caused by arboviruses, successful therapeutic studies with penicillin pointed to bacteria. This therapeutic approach was based on data from *Hellström,* reported by this author as early as 1951.

The second chapter in the history of the discovery of Lyme borreliosis was written in the USA. In the mid-1970s worried mothers of children with endemic arthritis in Old Lyme, Connecticut, contacted *Dr. Steere*, a rheumatologist at Yale University. Clinical and epidemiological studies led to the "rediscovery" of this clinical picture, which was now called "Lyme arthritis". *Dr. Steere* demonstrated the efficacy of antibiosis with the aid of randomized therapeutic studies. For a while, however, no causative organism could be identified until *Willy Burgdorfer* isolated a hitherto unclassified spirochete from an intestinal smear of *Ixodes dammini* ticks in Long Island, New York. Using immunological techniques he found that the serum of patients with Lyme arthritis contained antibodies which react specifically with the spirochete, and thus clarified the etiology of the disease. Not long after that, various research groups in the USA and Europe succeeded in isolating spirochetes from the skin, blood, and cerebrospinal fluid of patients with the disease. The spirochete, named after the person who first described it, was *Borrelia burgdorferi*. In the following decade the clinical pictures that had been discovered independently in Europe and the USA were shown to be a nosologically homogeneous infectious disease with a worldwide distribution. For historical reasons, the disease is referred to by several names:

- Lyme borreliosis
- Lyme disease
- Erythema migrans borreliosis
- Tick borreliosis, and
- *Borrelia burgdorferi* infection

> Lyme borreliosis has since become established as the internationally accepted term. If neurological and dermatological symptoms are present, the disease should be referred to as *neuroborreliosis* and *dermatoborreliosis* respectively.

Characteristics of the pathogen

2. Characteristics of the pathogen

2.1. Lyme borreliosis

2.1.1. Taxonomic classification

The genus *Borrelia* gets its name from the French microbiologist *A. Borrel*, and the species *Borrelia burgdorferi* is named after *Willy Burgdorfer*, who in 1982 was the first, together with *Alan Barbour*, to culture the organism which causes Lyme borreliosis. As a result of this work numerous long-familiar clinical pictures could now be clarified.

> *Borreliae* are gram-negative helical bacteria that grow under microaerophilic conditions. Because of their helical (spiral-shaped) appearance, they are classed as members of the Spirochaetaceae family, which is subdivided into the medically important genera Treponema, Leptospira and *Borrelia*.

The genus *Borrelia* can be split into the organisms which cause

- Relapsing fever
  - *B. recurrentis*
  - *B. duttoni*
  - *B. hermsii* etc.

and those which cause

- Lyme borreliosis
  - *B. burgdorferi* complex or
  - *B. burgdorferi* sensu lato (s.l.) , ☞ Fig. 2.1

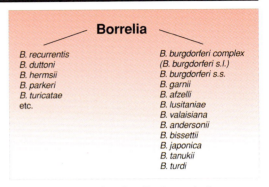

Fig. 2.1: Taxonomic classification of the genus *Borrelia*.

The organisms which cause Lyme borreliosis have so far been divided into 10 further genospecies or DNA groups with the aid of various molecular-genetic methods, such as:

- DNA-DNA hybridization
- RFLP (restriction fragment length polymorphism) analysis, and
- Sequencing of the "intergenic spacer" region of the rRNA operon (section of genetic material between the 5S rRNA gene and the 23S rRNA gene).

In Europe, however, human-pathogenic potential has only been firmly established for the following three genospecies:

- *B. burgdorferi* sensu stricto (s.s.)
- *B. garinii*, and
- *B. afzelii*,

Genotype	Vector	Geographic distribution	Pathogenicity
B. burgdorferi s.s.	Tick	North America/Europe	Pathogenic
B. garinii	Tick	Worldwide	Pathogenic
B. afzelii	Tick	Eurasia	Pathogenic
B. lusitaniae	Tick	Europe/North Africa	Unclear
B. valaisiana	Tick	Eurasia	Unclear
B. andersonii	Tick	North America	Unclear
B. bissettii	Tick	North America	Unclear
B. japonica	Tick	Asia	Unclear
B. tanukii	Tick	Asia	Unclear
B. turdi	Tick	Asia	Unclear

Table 2.1: Pathogenicity and classification of the *Borrelia burgdorferi* complex.

2.1. Lyme borreliosis

the other genospecies only having been isolated from ticks (☞ Table 2.1).

Using a further method of differentiation, the OspA/OspC serotyping system, the three genospecies

- *B. burgdorferi* s.s.
- *B. afzelii*, and
- *B. garinii*

can be subdivided into 7 OspA and 13 OspC serotypes (☞ Table 2.2).

Genospecies	OspA serotype	OspC serotype
B. burgdorferi s.s.	1	1-4
B. afzelii	2	5-8
B. garinii	3-7	8-13

Table 2.2: Distribution of OspA/OspC serotypes for the three human-pathogenic genospecies. OspC serotype 8 is found among *B. afzelii* isolates and also among *B. garinii* isolates, though it has not yet been detected among isolates of *B. burgdorferi* s.s..

This classification system uses the antigenic heterogeneity of the two lipoproteins on the outer membrane of *Borreliae*, OspA and OspC (☞ Fig. 2.5 and Sections 2.1.4. and 2.1.5.).

2.1.2. Morphology

In dark-field and phase-contrast microscopy *Borreliae* are recognizable by their irregular helical appearance. They are also noticeably elongated (10-30 µm) and very thin (0.2-0.25 µm) (☞ Fig. 2.2C and Figs. 6.1 and 6.4). Morphologically, moving from outside to inside, the following structural elements in the cross section of a *Borrelia* are encountered (☞ Fig. 2.2B and Fig. 2.3):

- 1. A 2-10 nm thick amorphous mucoid layer, also known as the **S-layer** or Surface layer
- 2. A very flexible **trilaminar membrane**
- 3. The **periplasmic space**
- 4. **Endoflagella**
- 5. A **protoplasmic cylinder**

The S-layer of *Borreliae* is characterized by a high level of instability and is very easily separated from the outer membrane. It does not show any substructural components in electron microscopy taken after negative staining. A further structural element is a highly flexible membrane, composed of three layers, within which (in the periplasmic space) are the endoflagella which enable the *Borreliae* to move and which entwine the protoplasmic cylinder like snakes along the entire length of the cell (☞ Fig. 2.2A).

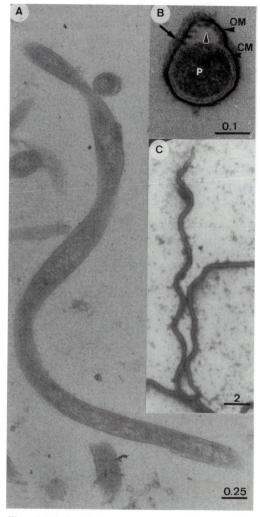

Figs. 2.2 A-C: Electron microscopy of *Borreliae* in longitudinal and cross section. **A**: Longitudinal thin-section of a *Borrelia*. **B**: Cross section profile of a *Borrelia*; CM: Cytoplasmic membrane, OM: Outer trilaminar membrane, P: Protoplasmic cylinder, endoflagella (9) indicated by tip of arrow and S-layer by arrow. **C**: Negative staining of *Borreliae*.

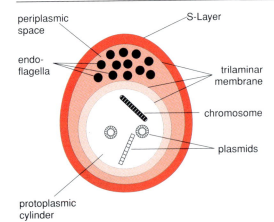

Fig. 2.3: Schematic structure of a *Borrelia* in cross section.

As with other *Borrelia* species and gram-negative bacteria, each endoflagellum consists of

- *a flagellar filament*
- *a flagellar hook*, and a
- *basal disk*.

Contraction of the flagella bundles which are attached subterminally at each end causes these pathogenic organisms to move in their characteristic rotating fashion. The number of endoflagella (3-18) depends on various factors:

- 1. The geographic origin of the isolate
- 2. The physiological state of the cell, and
- 3. The general conditions of culture (e.g. nutrient supply, pH)

The protoplasm cylinder, which is enclosed by the inner trilaminar membrane, contains the nucleoplasm, ribosomes, DNA-associated molecules, and other structures.

Borreliae also show two types of vesicle:

- 1. **Blebs** (eversions of the outer trilaminar membrane), and
- 2. **Gemmae** (up to 2 µm eversions of the outer membrane and protoplasmic membrane).

Blebs often form at the terminal end or laterally and are characteristic of dying cells. Serum-sensitive strains of *Borrelia* in particular develop numerous blebs after complement activation, and this is followed, after fairly lengthy incubation, by cell fragmentation (☞ Sections 4.1.1.4. and 4.1.2.1.).

Gemmae, which are associated with the outer membrane and located at the terminal end, make the *Borreliae* look as though they have spherical protuberance at the end. Their significance for pathogenesis in the human host is still unclear; however, given that plasmid DNA has been detected in the gemmae, it is conceivable that they might play a role in the alteration of virulence properties through plasmid loss or in the transfer of genetic material (☞ Section 2.1.4.).

2.1.3. Culture conditions

Borreliae can only be cultured *in vitro* in a very nutrient-rich medium supplemented with amino acids, vitamins, bovine serum albumin, and rabbit serum (modified Barbour-Stoenner-Kelly (BSK) medium) (☞ Section 6.1.3.1.2.). The optimum temperature for growth is 30-34°C. The generation time under cultural microaerophilic conditions is 7-20 h, cell concentrations of 10^6-10^8/ml being achievable with adapted laboratory strains.

Defined clones are obtained by microdilution techniques or by culture on solid media over a period of 2-5 weeks.

2.1.4. Molecular biology aspects

A characteristic of *Borreliae* which sets them apart from other microorganisms is that they have a **linear** chromosome and in addition up to 20 different **linear** and **circular** plasmids, also known as **minichromosomes**. Toward the end of 1997 the complete gene sequence of the *Borrelia* chromosome and of nine linear and two circular plasmids of the B31 strain of *B. burgdorferi* s.s. was published for the first time.

853 genes on the chromosome — which consists of 910725 bp (GC-content 28.6 %) — code, among other things, for proteins involved in:

- DNA replication, transcription, and translation
- The repair system and recombination
- Transport, nutrient uptake and energy metabolism
- Motility and chemotaxis
- The regulation of gene expression

The absence of genes coding for the synthesis of amino acids, fatty acids, cofactors, and nucleotides explains why culture calls for the use of a complex, serum-supplemented cell culture medium. Furthermore, since *Borreliae* are chemoorganotrophic microaerophilic microorganisms, they need to obtain their biochemical energy (ATP) from substrate phosphorylation that takes place in the cytoplasm, particularly as there are no genes which code for the components of respiratory chain phosphorylation. Pyruvate, which is one of the most important intermediate compounds in metabolism and enables the cell to use released energy for anabolism and for the maintenance of vital function, is probably obtained mainly from glucose the primary substrate, by glycolysis. *Borreliae* also lack other enzymes needed for the tricarboxylic acid cycle or oxidative phosphorylation. Since the capacity of their metabolism components is so limited, they can only survive if they have a host organism to ensure their supply of nutrients.

Extrachromosomal elements (plasmids) are not unusual among microorganisms. However, the fact that *Borreliae* can have as many as 20 different (linear or circular) plasmids sets them clearly apart from other bacteria. Even among individual isolates there are tremendous variations in the number and size (9-70 kb) of the plasmids. After electrophoretic separation of isolated plasmids in agarose gel, each isolate shows a characteristic plasmid profile that can be used as an additional differentiation parameter. The *B. garinii* isolate PSth, for example, has up to 6 clearly identifiable plasmid bands (☞ Fig. 2.4, No. 8).

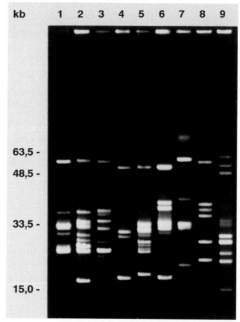

Fig. 2.4: Gel-electrophoretic separation of plasmids of various strains of *Borrelia* by PFGE. Ba strain FEM1 (1), Ba strain PKo (2), Ba strain EB1 (3), Bb strain B31 (4), Bb strain 297 (5), Bb strain PKa1 (6), Bg strain G1 (7), Bg strain PSth (8), Bg strain A76S (9); **Ba**: *B. afzelii*, **Bb**: *B. burgdorferi* s.s., **Bg**: *B. garinii*.

However, in *Borrelia*, in contrast to many other bacteria, plasmids are found only in a **single** copy or in a few copies per chromosome in the cell. Repeated passaging of the cells over a prolonged period often results in loss of the plasmids. The associated changes in the cells' protein and antigen profile can lead to a loss of infectivity. It is therefore presumed that plasmid-encoded proteins (antigens) in particular are substantially responsible for virulence.

Only 16 % of the total 430 open reading frames (longer DNA segments uninterrupted by termination codons, which code for proteins) of the 11 sequenced plasmids of the *B. burgdorferi* strain B31 could be assigned to known proteins. They include:

- Various lipoproteins (OspA-D)
- Porins
- Decorin-binding proteins
- Enzymes for purine synthesis and
- Various antigens

Protein	Apparent molecular weight (kDa)	Genetic location	Plasmid size (kb)	Immunogenicity in human host
OspA	31-33	Linear plasmid	54	Yes
OspB	34-36	Linear plasmid	54	Yes
OspC	20-23	Circular plasmid	26	Yes
OspD	28	Linear plasmid	38	No
OspE	19	Linear plasmid	45	No
OspF	26	Linear plasmid	45	No
EppA	18	Circular plasmid	9	No
Flagellin (p41)	41	Chromosomal	-	Yes
Oms66 (p66)	66	Chromosomal	-	Yes
p83/100	80-100	Chromosomal	-	Yes
BmpA (p39)	39	Chromosomal	-	Yes
p18	18	Plasmid	?	Yes

Table 2.3: Genetic location of various membrane proteins and their immunogenic significance. **Osp**: Outer surface protein, **EppA**: Exported protein A, **Oms**: Outer membrane-spanning protein, **Bmp**: Basic membrane protein

Many of these membrane (lipo)proteins are immunogenic and induce a strong immune response, and are thus of particular importance for diagnostics (☞ Table 2.3 and Section 6.1.3.5.).

Since a change of the host leads to drastic ecological changes, *Borreliae* must be able to adapt their biosynthesis to their new environment within a very short time and so must be capable of coordinated gene expression.

The temperature-dependent gene regulation best studied in *Borreliae* to date relates to the two outer membrane proteins OspA and OspC. Surface-expressed lipoprotein OspA is detectable in *Borreliae* before the tick engorged, though not after it has stopped doing so (downregulation of OspA). At temperatures below 24°C there is little or no expression of OspC in the tick midgut. When blood flows into the tick's midgut, the temperature increases, inducing expression of OspC (upregulation of OspC), which is then detectable on the membrane surface. This explains the very weak immune response to OspA and the very strong immune response to OspC (☞ Section 6.1.3.2.1.). Other proteins are expressed only in the tick and/or the human host and not under culture conditions. One example is the membrane protein EppA encoded on circular plasmid cp9 (☞ Table 2.3).

Surface-protein modification may be correlated with poorer growth *in vitro* and changes in binding to endothelial cells or in sensitivity to complement.

2.1.5. Antigen structure and antigenic diversity of *B. burgdorferi* s.l.

After electrophoretic separation of whole-cell lysates with SDS-PAGE it is possible to identify more than 30 different protein bands (☞ Fig. 2.5). Irrespective of their geographic or biological origin, *Borreliae* have two main protein components with constant molecular weights of 41 kDa (p41 or flagellin) and 60 kDa (HSP60). Flagellin has serotype-specific epitopes as well as cross-reacting epitopes, whereas the HSP60 protein shows a high degree of cross-reactivity with other bacteria.

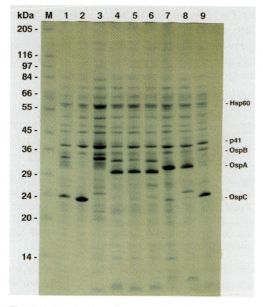

Fig. 2.5: Electrophoretic separation of ultrasonicate extracts of *Borrelia* strains by Tricin-SDS-PAGE. Ba strain FEM1 (1), Ba strain Pko (2), Ba strain MMS (3), Bb strain B31 (4), Bb strain 297 (5), Bb strain PKa1 (6), Bg strain G1 (7), Bg strain PSth (8), Bg strain A76S (9); **Ba**: *B. afzelii*, **Bb**: *B. burgdorferi* s.s., **Bg**: *B. garinii*. M: molecular weight markers.

Three other characteristic bands in SDS-PAGE represent membrane lipoproteins with varying molecular weights, of 31-33 kDa (OspA), 34-36 kDa (OspB), and 20-23 kDa (OspC) (☞ Fig. 2.5). In culture, European *Borrelia* strains generally express OspA and/or OspC, but only rarely OspB. The protein profile of North American strains of *B. burgdorferi* s.s. shows a uniform band for OspA and a variable one for OspB; OspC is seldom present. The two membrane proteins OspA and OspC are currently regarded as the **principal candidates for the development of a successful vaccine** (☞ Section 8.2.).

The only *Borrelia* antigens that have been well characterized immunologically are membrane proteins, such as:

- p83/100
- Oms66 (p66)
- BmpA (p39)
- HSP60 (p60)
- p18
- OspD
- OspE and
- OspF

Interestingly, most of these immunogenically active proteins are plasmid-encoded (☞ Table 2.3). Plasmid loss thus necessarily leads to a change in antigen structure, which increases the diversity of the immune response and favors persistence of the causative organism (☞ Section 4.1.2.2.)

2.2. Tick-borne encephalitis (TBE)

2.2.1. Taxonomic classification and structure of the TBE virus

Taxonomically, the TBE virus (syn. tick-borne encephalitis virus; TBEV) belongs to the Flavivirus genus, which can be divided into approximately 100 different serotypes. In the Eurasian region two subtypes of TBE are distinguished:

- 1. Subtype 1, the *European* subtype, the organism which causes Central European encephalitis (CEE) and

- 2. Subtype 2, the *Far Eastern* subtype, the organism which causes Russian tick-borne encephalitis (RTBE)

The close relation between the two subtypes can be seen from the high degree (up to 96 %) of amino acid sequence homology.

The viruses are transmitted through **bites of infected ticks** of the genus *I. ricinus* (subtype 1) or *I. persulcatus* (subtype 2; ☞ Section 3.1.1.) or other infected arthropods (e.g. mosquitoes). The most important human-pathogenic viruses, other than the TBE virus, are the numerous flaviviruses related to the TBE virus:

- Yellow fever virus
- Japanese encephalitis virus
- Dengue viruses

or viruses of the Togaviridae family.

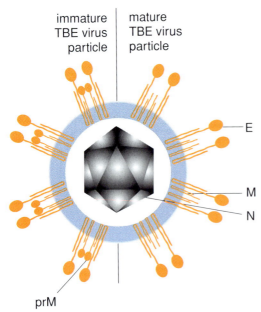

Fig. 2.6: Schematic model of mature and immature TBE virions. **E**: Glycoprotein E, **M**: Glycoprotein M (modified after translation, only present in mature virions), **prM**: Glycoprotein prM (only present in immature virions), **N**: Nucleocapsid (according to Heinz and Mandl, 1993, modified).

Structurally, the TBE virus is no different from other flaviviruses; its genomic RNA is infectious, which, with the capsid protein (protein C), forms an icosahedral nucleocapsid. The protein coat surrounding the capsid consists mainly of glycoprotein E and, in **mature** virus particles, of the membrane-associated M protein (☞ Fig. 2.6). The total diameter is about 50 nm.

2.2.2. Molecular biology aspects

All flaviviruses possess single-stranded RNA of positive polarity (+/ssRNA) consisting of approximately 11 000 nucleotides. This acts as the only viral mRNA in the infected cell, so that reverse transcription of RNA to give cDNA is no longer necessary because of its polarity. As far as organization of the genetic material is concerned, the viral genome is clearly divided into two parts: the sequences of structural proteins (C= core, prM/M= membrane protein, and E= envelope) are located in the first quarter and the sequences of all other (nonstructural) proteins (NS1, NS2A, NS2B, NS3, NS4A, NS4B and NS5) are located at the 3´-end

(☞ Fig. 2.7). At the 5´- and 3´-terminations the TBE virus genome is flanked by noncoding regions (NCR), which exert important regulatory functions during the viral replication cycle through the formation of secondary RNA structures.

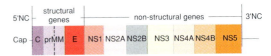

Fig. 2.7: Schematic diagram of the genetic organization of the TBE virus. **C**: Cytoplasmic protein, **prM/M**: Glycoprotein prM/M, **E**: Glycoprotein E (envelope protein), **NS**: Nonstructural protein, **NC**: 5´- and 3´-noncoding regions, Cap: Cap structure of the RNA (according to Heinz and Mandl, 1993, modified)

Unlike togaviruses, whose RNA codes only for nonstructural proteins, flaviviruses synthesize all proteins — both structural and nonstructural — from this single positive strand. A polyprotein consisting of around 3414 amino acids is formed. After translocation of this polyprotein through the host cell's endoplasmic reticulum (ER) membrane, proteins prM (precursor to M), E, NS1, and NS4B remain in the lumen of the ER until the viral polyprotein translocation process is complete. Further posttranslational steps then take place in the lumen of the ER or the cytoplasm. Both cellular and virus-specific endopeptidases are involved in these cotranslational or posttranslational processing reactions.

2.2.3. Antigen structure of the TBE virus

The most important antigen of the TBE virus is protein E, which is involved in receptor binding and activates the fusion between the virus and the human host cell. It is a strong immunogen and, after active immunization, gives protection comparable with that afforded by inactivated virions. This glycoprotein consists of three domains A, B, and C. Domain A is highly conserved and plays an important role in fusion. Neutralizing antibodies and also hemagglutination- and fusion-inhibiting antibodies bind to domain B, the most important determinant of virus particle virulence. No specific function has yet been assigned to domain C. Mutations in other regions outside domain B also change the pathogenicity and are consequently important for the control of virulence and attenuation. During the maturation of the virus particle, complexing with glycoprotein prM protects protein E from irreversible conformational change and aggregation, ensuring a high level of virulence (and thus survival) of the virus particle. At low pH values, such as are found in the vesicles, conformational rearrangements occur — particularly in domain A. At the same time, however, this low pH is needed for fusion and endocytosis and for the proteolytic cleavage of prM to form protein M.

References

Burgdorfer W., Barbour A.G., Hayes S.F., Grunwaldt E., Davis J.P. (1982). Lyme disease - a tick-borne spirochetosis? Science 216: 1317-1319

Carrol J.A., Gherardini F.C. (1996). Membrane protein variations associated with in vitro passage of *Borrelia burgdorferi*. Infect. Immun. 64: 392-398

De Silva A.M., Fikrig E. (1997). *Borrelia burgdorferi* genes selectively expressed in ticks and mammals. Parasitol. today 13: 267-270

Foretz M., Postic D., Baranton G. (1997). Phylogenetic analysis of *Borrelia burgdorferi* sensu stricto by arbitrarily primed PCR and pulse-fieled gel electrophoresis. Int. J. Syst. Bacteriol. 47: 11-18

Fraser C.M., Casjens S., Huang W.M., Sutton G.G., Clayton R., Lathigra R., White O., Ketchum K.A., Dodson R., Hickey E.K., Gwinn M., Dougherty B., Tomb J.F., Fleischmann R.D., Richardson D., Peterson J., Kerlavage A.R., Quackenbush J., Salzberg S., Hanson M., van Vugt R., Palmer N., Adams M.D., Gocayne J., Weidman J., Utterback T., Watthey L., McDonald L., Artiach P., Bowman Ch., Garland S., Fujii C., Cotton M.D., Horst K., Roberst K., Hatch B., Smith H.O., Venter J.C. (1997). Genomic sequence of a Lyme disease spirochaete, *Borrelia burgdorferi*. Nature 390: 580-586

Hayes S.F., Burgdorfer W. (1993). *Ultrastructure of Borrelia burdorferi* in: Aspects of Lyme borreliosis, Weber K. Burdorfer W (Eds.) Springer-Verlag, Berlin Heidelberg 29-43

Heinz F.X., Mandl C.W. (1993). The molecular biology of tick-borne encephalitis virus. APMIS 101: 735-745

Monath T.P. (1990). Flaviviruses. In : Virology, Fields B. N. (Ed.) Raven Press, New York 763-814

Montgomery R.R., Malawista S.E., Feen K.J.M., Bockenstedt L. (1996). Direct demonstration of antigenic substitution of *Borrelia burgdorferi* ex vivo: exploration of the paradox of the early immune response to outer surface protein A and C in Lyme disease. J. Exp. Med. 183: 261-269

Preac-Mursic V., Wilske B. (1993). Biology of *Borrelia burgdorferi* in: Aspects of Lyme borreliosis, Weber K., Burdorfer W. (Eds.) Springer-Verlag, Berlin Heidelberg 44-58

Schwan T.G., Piesman J., Golde W.T., Dolan M.C., Rosa P.A. (1995). Induction of an outer surface protein on *Borrelia burgdorferi* during tick feeding. Proc. Natl. Acad. Sci. 92: 2909-2913

Suk K., Das S., Sun W., Jwang B., Barthold S.W., Flavell R.A., Fikrig E. (1995). *Borrelia burgdorferi* genes selectively expressed in the infected host. Proc. Natl. Acad. Sci. USA 92: 4269-4273

Wilske B., Preac-Mursic V., Göbel U.B., Graf B., Jauris S., Soutchek E., Schwab E., Zumstein G. (1993). An OspA serotyping system for *Borrelia burgdorferi* based on reactivity with monoclonal antibodies and OspA sequence analysis. J. Clin. Microbiol. 31: 340-350

Wilske B., Jauris-Heipke S., Lobentanzer R., Pradel I., Preac-Mursic V., Rössler D., Soutchek E., Johnson R.C. (1993). Phenotypic analysis of outer surface protein C (OspC) of *Borrelia burgdorferi* sensu lato by monoclonal antibodies: relationship to genospecies and OspA serotype. J. Clin. Microbiol. 33: 103-109

Xu Y., Johnson R.C. (1995). Analysis and comparison of plasmid profiles of *Borrelia burgdorferi* sensu lato strains. J. Clin. Microbiol. 33: 2679-2685

Xu Y., Kodner C., Coleman L., Johnson R.C. (1996). Correlation of plasmids with infectivity of *Borrelia burgdorferi* sensu stricto type strain B31. Infect. Immun. 64: 3870-3876

Tick ecology and epidemiology

3. Tick ecology and epidemiology

3.1. Tick ecology

To understand the endemic occurrence of Lyme borreliosis and TBE, it is essential to know something of the ecology of their principal vector: ticks.

3.1.1. Ticks — a general introduction

Being hematophagous ectoparasites, ticks must suck the blood of vertebrates in order to live. Zoologically, they belong to the class of Arachnida (subphylum Chelicerata), together with spiders and scorpions. There are two families of ticks:
- Soft-bodied ticks (*Argasidae*) and
- Hard-bodied ticks (*Ixodidae*)

Soft ticks live mainly in warm climates; consuming their meal of blood within a matter of hours. Hard ticks have a wider geographic distribution, which in some instances extends into subarctic regions, though most species prefer temperate climates; feeding extends over a number of days and can go on for as long as 3 weeks.

However, ticks are important not only as blood-sucking parasites, but also as vectors (carriers) of pathogenic microorganisms, including:
- The world's commonest form of endemic encephalitis — tick-borne encephalitis (causative organism: TBE virus; ☞ Section 2.2)
- Japanese encephalitis (causative organism: *Flavivirus*)
- Rocky Mountain spotted fever (causative organism: *Rickettsia rickettsii*)
- Ehrlichiosis (causative organism: *Ehrlichia phagocytophila*)
- Tularemia (causative organism: *Francisella tularensis*)
- Lyme borreliosis (causative organism: *Borrelia burgdorferi*)

> In Central Europe the hard-bodied tick *Ixodes ricinus*, generally known as the 'wood tick', is an extremely important vector in the transmission of Lyme borreliosis, caused by the bacterium *B. burgdorferi*, and viral TBE.

3.1.2. Ixodes ricinus

The hard tick *Ixodes (I.) ricinus* is indigenous to the whole of Europe (except Iceland) between sea level and altitudes of around 2000 m, and prefers locations with high humidity and moderate temperatures. The sites most favorable to its development are forest margins, clearings, and path edges in dense deciduous or mixed forests with herbaceous or grassy undergrowth. It used to be found only in areas dominated by arable farming; however, changes in the way in which land is used in gardens and parks have meant an increase in tick populations in these locations as well.

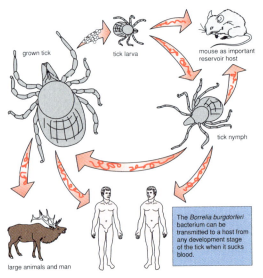

Fig. 3.1: Life cycle of the hard tick Ixodes ricinus and transmission of the organism that causes Lyme borreliosis (with kind permission of Dr. Bösebeck, HMR Deutschland).

The ticks live for up to 6 years, during which they pass through three developmental stages (☞ Figs. 3.1 and 3.2c+d):
- Larva
- Nymph
- Sexually mature tick

March to October is considered to be the period of peak tick activity, diurnal fluctuations being the norm (maxima in the morning and evening, minimum in the hours around midday). Sexually mature females are an elongated oval shape and, unlike the males, do not have a rigid chitinous scutellum.

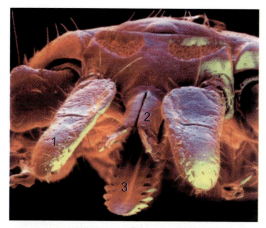

a

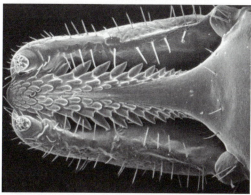

b

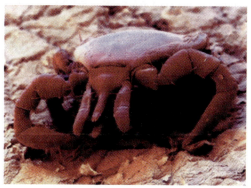

c

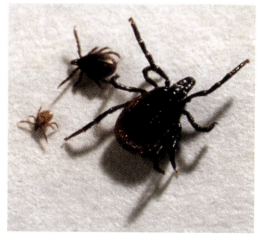

d

Figs. 3.2a-d: a: Dorsal view of the mouthparts of adult Ixodes ricinus. Moving from the outside in, the pairs of pedipalps (1) and chelicerae (2) are encountered, and also the dorsally flattened hypostome (3) (with kind permission of Chiron Behring GmbH); **b:** ventral view of the mouthparts of a female Ixodes ricinus. The hypostome can be seen to be a flattened part, dentate only on the ventral side. The ventral view also shows the palps, which do not penetrate the skin of the victim (☞ Fig. 8.1a) (with kind permission of Prof. Matuschka, Pathology Institute, Charité, Berlin); **c:** Adult tick; **d:** Developmental stages of the tick (with kind permission of Prof. Matuschka, Pathology Institute, Charité, Berlin).

Their body length is given as approximately 2.4-4.8 mm; however, the absence of a chitin scutum means that it can increase to 12 to nearly 30 mm after a meal of blood. The bodies of nymphs (fasting: 1.2 mm; engorged: 2 mm) are shorter than those of larvae (fasting: 0.6 mm; engorged: up to 1.25 mm). Sexually mature ticks are ready to mate in the fall. The male dies shortly after mating; the female lays up to several thousand eggs early the following spring. The six-legged larvae hatch out a few weeks after laying. They feed on the blood of their hosts, mainly small rodents, e.g. mice of the genera *Apodemus* (yellow-necked field mouse, wood mouse), *Clethrionomys* (red-backed mouse) and *Peromyscus* (white-footed mouse), but occasionally also birds and larger mammals. They hibernate among leaves or in the top soil layer. The larvae grow during the hibernation phase, and, as soon as the ground temperature reaches about 5-7°C in spring, they become active again as eight-legged nymphs. The nymphs too feed on the blood of various hosts, mainly small mammals (e.g. hedgehogs or squirrels) and birds which spend relatively much time on the ground (thrush, songthrush). After its meal of blood the nymph leaves the host and, after growing and molting, reaches the adult stage. The sexually mature tick is also known as an imago. After a maturation period lasting days to weeks, and possibly even months, the adult female tick looks for further hosts on which to feed, up until fall — it climbs vegetation of up to 1.50 m in height and attaches itself to new hosts as they brush past, requiring only a fraction of a second of direct contact for the transfer. The main hosts at this stage are the roe deer (*Capreolus capreolus*) and red deer (*Cervus elaphus*) and other large mammals, such as man and domesticated animals. The ticks, which do not have eyes, locate an appropriate host with a sensory organ known as Haller's organ, which is used to ascertain the CO_2 concentration of ambient air and to detect thermal radiation and movement in the surrounding vegetation caused by a passing host. Once on the host, the tick may spend several hours looking for suitable feeding sites — the preferred location of which varies, depending on the growth stage of the tick and species of the host — with the aid of sensory setae. Then, within a matter of minutes, it pierces the cutis and subcutis of their victim (ticks do not *bite*) with its piercing-sucking mouthparts (☞ Figs. 3.2a+b), sucking blood for periods ranging between several days and 3 weeks, anesthetizing the puncture site with its saliva. Mating between the sexually mature male and female ticks takes place on the host. The ticks then drop off into surrounding vegetation and females look for a suitable laying site on the ground.

Ants, lizards, birds, and shrews are natural tick antagonists. In addition, ticks are parasitized by parasitic wasps, which lay their eggs on them, the ticks serving as a source of food for the hatched wasps.

3.2. Epidemiology

Epidemiology is the study of the frequency (prevalence and incidence) and distribution of diseases and their causes and risk factors in population groups (compared with the population as a whole or with other groups) and, of their course and social and economic consequences. It also involves investigations of the value of diagnostic methods and preventive measures and the recording and presentation of disease statistics. Since several of the above-mentioned aspects are considered at length in particular sections of this book, below we shall deal mainly with the frequency and distribution of tick-borne diseases.

3.2.1. Lyme borreliosis

Lyme borreliosis is the commonest tick-borne zoonosis in Europe and North America. It is estimated that in Germany there are perhaps as many as 60 000 new cases per year. It is not a notifiable disease and so no exact data are available. It is caused by the human-pathogenic spirochete *B. burgdorferi* s.l., which is divided into three species:

- *B. burgdorferi* s.s., which is found mainly in Europe and North America,

- *B. afzelii*, which is found chiefly in Europe, and

- *B. garinii*, which is found predominantly in Europe and in the temperate regions of Asia.

In addition, all species show molecular polymorphism, manifested in a heterogenicity of the surface-proteins. This is important for the immunological responses of the infected person, for diagnosis with serological test methods, and for the clinical manifestations, which differ from region to region. For example, acrodermatitis chronica atrophicans and neuroborreliosis are more frequent in Europe, whereas Lyme arthritis is more frequent in the USA (☞ Section 5.1.2.).

Tick species	Geographic distribution
I. ricinus	Europe
I. persulcatus	Eastern Europe, Asia
I. dammini/ scapularis	Midwestern, northeast and southeast USA, Canada
I. pacificus	Pacific coast of Central and North America [from Baja (Mexico), through California (USA), to British Columbia (Canada)] and Midwestern USA (Nevada, Utah, Idaho)

Table 3.1: Geographic distribution of the commonest B. burgdorferi-carrying ticks

3.2. Epidemiology

B. burgdorferi is carried by various species of the hard-bodied tick family (☞ Table 3.1), depending on the geographic location, though also (rarely) by other arthropods such as mosquitoes, horseflies, and other tick families (see above). The bacterium is ingested with blood sucked from the competent host and then remains in the tick's digestive tract or migrates, via hemolymph, to the salivary glands and other organs, including in particular the ovaries of the female tick. Transovarian transmission to offspring of the affected female is thus also a possibility. *B. burgdorferi* is transmitted to a fresh host when the tick again sucks blood, generally after about 24-48 h, either through regurgitation from the digestive tract or by introduction of infected saliva into the host's bloodstream while the tick is feeding. The risk of infection can therefore be reduced by the prompt removal of ticks.

The hosts of *I. ricinus* can be divided into two groups:

- One group serves mainly as a blood reservoir for tick development. The roe deer for example, though a primary host of the adult ticks, is not a competent reservoir for *B. burgdorferi*. Nevertheless, given the rapid and focal endemic spread of Lyme borreliosis in Sweden and the northwestern USA, the spread of infected ticks by a spreading population of increasing numbers of roe deer is assumed to be one of the causes. In addition to this, birds spread the disease over great distances and heights, creating new regions of infection.
- The importance of the other host group, on the other hand, is as a carrier reservoir for *B. burgdorferi*: e.g. small rodents (mice), in which *B. burgdorferi* can survive for years without provoking any symptoms. In Europe there are 8 mammals considered to be capable of acting as competent host for *B. burgdorferi*: the mice *Apodemus* (A.) *sylvaticus*, *A. flavicollis* and *A. agrarius*, *Sorex* (S.) *araneus* and *S. minutus*, and *Clethrionomys glareolus* and the hares *Lepus* (L.) *europaeus* and *L. timidus*.

> The estimates of the tick infection levels with *B. burgdorferi* vary according to region and growth stage:
> - Nymphs:
>   - Switzerland 5-34 %
>   - Germany 3-26 %
>   - USA (north-east) 25-50 %
>   - Sweden < 15 %
>   - Slovenia 4 %
> - Sexually mature tick:
>   - Germany 11-34 %
>   - USA (north-east) > 50 %
>   - Sweden 13-29 %
>   - Slovenia 23 %
>   - Russia: up to 30 % of I. ricinus and up to 50-60 % of I. persulcatus
>
> In TBE areas ticks may be infected simultaneously with *Borreliae* and with the TBE virus.

In contrast to TBE, which occurs endemically, no regions of endemic occurrence or natural foci of *Borrelia*-infected ticks can be discerned in Germany and neighboring European countries. Each year tens of thousands of cases of Lyme borreliosis are reported outside Germany across Europe. A similar picture is seen in the USA (1994: 13 043 cases), though there the disease sometimes occurs endemically, particularly in the northeastern parts (Massachusetts to Maryland), the Midwest (Wisconsin and Minnesota), and the Pacific coast (California and Oregon). Lyme borreliosis also occurs in the Baltic, the region of the former USSR, in Israel, China, Japan, Australia, South Africa, and on the South American continent.

Region	Serological prevalence (%)	Incidence (per 100 000 inhabitants each year)
Sweden	7-29	69
USA (Connecticut)	3	41
USA (elsewhere)	No data	3.3
Austria	3.8-7.7	No data
Italy	15.5-36.3	17
Switzerland	10.7	No data
Germany	3-17	22
Belgium	2.9	No data
UK	1-7	No data
Ireland	9.75	No data
Lithuania	4-32	No data
Croatia	8	No data
Slovenia	No data	114-137
St. Petersburg	7-16	3.9

Table 3.2: Epidemiological data on Lyme borreliosis for selected countries. The data come from various published studies and, in each instance, relate only to limited parts of the countries concerned. In contrast to the situation for TBE, no exact 'country' data are available for Lyme borreliosis.

Lyme borreliosis is encountered mainly in the months of July to September, in line with the periods of high tick activity (☞ Section 5. and Fig. 5.4). Chronic Lyme borreliosis can be observed all year round. The mean age of the patients is 44 years, more men being affected by the disease than women. 30-40 % of patients recall having been bitten by a tick. The serological-prevalence and incidence data vary considerably according to geographic location (☞ Table 3.2).

Seroepidemiological studies have shown the serological prevalence of Lyme borreliosis to be distinctly higher in high-risk groups such as forestry workers, cross-country runners, and agricultural laborers — prevalence of increased serum antibody titer 20-47 % versus 3-17 % in the normal population. Four weeks after a tick bite the level of clinically manifest Lyme borreliosis, in the Tyrol for example, was roughly 4 %, while the level of seroconversion was 20 %. Overall, the risk of developing Lyme borreliosis after a tick bite was calculated as about 1-5 %. In elevated-risk groups such as forestry officials, forestry workers, hunters, agricultural laborers, and cross-country runners, the likelihood of developing the disease is several times higher on account of their increased exposure to ticks.

3.2.2. Tick-borne encephalitis (TBE)

The TBE virus, the organism that causes tick-borne encephalitis (TBE) in Eurasia, is a spherical (icosahedral) capsid surrounded by a lipid membrane, with a diameter of approximately 500 Å. It is a flavivirus of the Flaviviridae family (☞ Section 2.2.). The following two subtypes are distinguished:

- Subtype 1, the organism which causes Central European encephalitis (CEE), and
- Subtype 2, the organism which causes Russian tick-borne encephalitis (RTBE) (☞ Fig. 3.3).

In addition to these, in various parts of the world there are inflammatory diseases involving the central nervous system (meningitis, encephalitis, meningoencephalitis) which are caused either by various flaviviruses related to the TBE virus and carried by arthropods (Dengue fever, yellow fever, St. Louis encephalitis, Japanese encephalitis, West Nile encephalitis, Murray Valley encephalitis) or by viruses of the Togaviridae family (Alphavirus: Eastern, Western, and Venezuelan equine encephalitis) and Bunyaviridae family (Bunyavirus: California encephalitis). Some 100 serotypes of the TBE complex have been isolated in the world as a whole. The most important vector of the TBE virus in Germany is considered to be I. ricinus, while subtype 2, the eastern variant (RTBE virus), is carried by the tick I. persulcatus.

In Europe, extensive areas of endemic occurrence can be distinguished for TBE, in contrast to the case of Lyme borreliosis; in these areas approximately 0.1-4.5 % of all ticks are infected with TBE viruses (☞ Figs. 3.4 and 3.5). Regions of endemic disease, which are also described as active natural foci, are circumscribed areas in which there have been several cases of TBE each year for a number of consecutive years (☞ Table 3.3 and Fig. 3.5)

3.2. Epidemiology

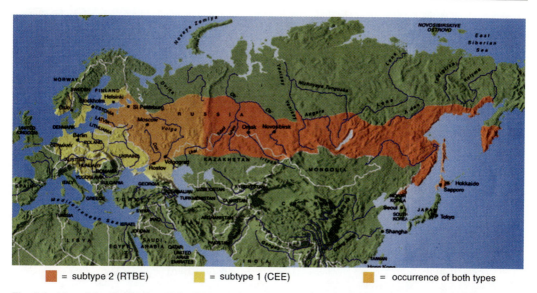

■ = subtype 2 (RTBE)　　■ = subtype 1 (CEE)　　■ = occurrence of both types

Fig. 3.3: Map of the distribution of the TBE subtypes (with kind permission of Chiron Behring GmbH).

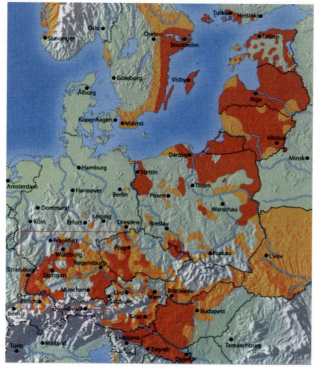

Fig. 3.4: Endemic TBE regions in northern Europe. **Red**: High-risk regions (high risk of developing the disease, several or many cases of TBE in the last few years; **Orange**: Low risk of developing the disease, few or no cases of TBE in the last few years. Sources: Germany: evaluation by Prof. Roggendorf and associates, 4th Potsdam Symposium (1997); Dr. G. Dobler, Mitteilungen der Bayrischen Gesellschaft für Immun-, Tropenmedizin und Impfwesen e. V., Vol. 14, No. 5, November 1997; PD Dr. R. Kaiser, Ärzteblatt Baden-Würtemberg 4/1997. Other European countries: data from the WHO and information from hygiene and/or university institutes of the various countries (with kind permission of Chiron Behring GmbH).

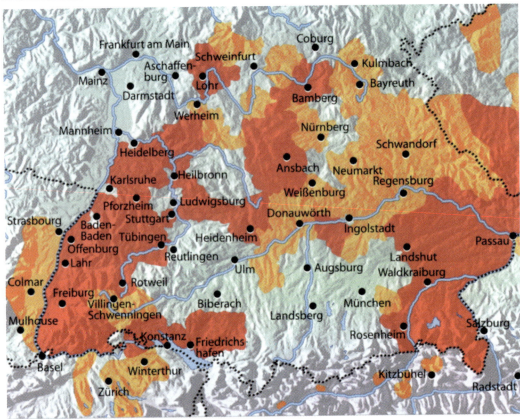

Fig. 3.5: Endemic TBE regions in southern Germany. **Red**: High-risk regions (high risk of developing the disease, several or many cases of TBE in the last few years; **Orange**: Low risk of developing the disease, few or no cases of TBE in the last few years. Sources: Germany: evaluation by Prof. Roggendorf and associates, 4th Potsdam Symposium (1997); Dr. G. Dobler, Mitteilungen der Bayrischen Gesellschaft für Immun-, Tropenmedizin und Impfwesen e. V., Vol. 14, No. 5, November 1997; PD Dr. R. Kaiser, Ärzteblatt Baden-Würtemberg 4/1997. Other European countries: data from the WHO and information from hygiene institutes and/or university institutes of the various countries (with kind permission of Chiron Behring GmbH).

Natural foci are characterized by particular climatic characteristics (mean annual temperature, sufficient atmospheric humidity) and geological conditions (soil type, vegetation), high population densities of carrier arthropods and their hosts, and their immunity status.

Country	Regions with an increased risk of TBE infection
Albania*	Throughout the country
Bosnia*	Northern parts of the country
Germany	Mainly the eastern parts of Bavaria, mainly the southwestern parts of Baden-Württemberg, a few small natural foci outside these states
Estonia*	Throughout the country
Finland	In the south-west, on Baltic islands
France	Alsace
Greece	Small natural focus near Thessaloniki
CIS*	Russia: throughout the country, including the Asiatic part, natural foci in Belarus, Ukraine (data in some instances incomplete or absent)
Italy	Two natural foci in the north (area surrounding Florence/Trieste)
Croatia*	Northern parts of the country
Latvia*	Throughout the country
Lithuania*	Throughout the country
Norway	Coastal areas in the south-west
Austria	River plains along the Danube; parts of Lower Austria, Carinthia, Styria, Burgenland
Poland*	North-east, south
Sweden	Southeast coast, west of Stockholm, Baltic islands
Switzerland	North — particularly the Lake Constance area, Rhine valley
Serbia*	West of Belgrade
Slovak Republic*	Throughout the country at less than 600 m above sea level, mainly the south-west
Slovenia*	Northern parts of the country
Czech Republic*	Mainly the river plains around Prague
Hungary	North, Lake Balaton, west of the Danube

* = Transmission of the disease in foodstuffs (sheep's milk and goats' milk) has been observed.

Table 3.3: Natural foci (= regions of endemic occurrence, with an increased risk of infection) of TBE in Europe.

These maps of endemic disease regions do not mean that there is no risk of infection outside them, since the virus may be brought into previously virus-free regions by animals carrying infected ticks (such as birds of the order Falconiformes or roe deer). People who live in areas of endemic occurrence and are exposed to tick bites during work and/or recreation, or people who travel to such areas, e.g. for leisure pursuits (hiking, camping), run a particularly high risk of TBE. The results of studies from the German state of Baden-Württemberg, with highly active pockets of endemic disease, show that nearly 90 % of the cases that occurred here were during leisure time. For natural foci in Germany the mean relative risk of viral infection as a result of tick bites has been given as 1:50 to 1:1000; the risk of infection in other countries in central Europe and, particularly in eastern Europe (Austria, Hungary, Slovak Republic) is distinctly greater, 1 in every 25-500 ticks in the regions of endemic occurrence being a virus carrier. According to recent studies the contagion index, i.e. the risk of developing disease as a result of infection, in Germany is 30-50 % (☞ Section 5.2.1.); the number of affected men is more than double that of affected women.

Mortality from subtype 1 (the western subtype) is given as approximately 0.5-2 %; the disease generally has a milder course in children than in adults. Subtype 2, the eastern subtype, is characterized by distinctly higher (two-figure) percentage mortality; however, more precise data are lacking. Reports concerning the current incidence of TBE in Germany put the number of cases of new infection at between 70-100 and 1000 per year, though this is difficult to confirm statistically.

> Although, according to § 3, paragraph 2 of BSeuchG [German Federal Infectious Diseases Act], TBE is a legally notifiable disease in the Federal Republic of Germany, hardly any valid statistics are available from the relevant health authorities.

There is a degree of uncertainty here, because the statistics include infections that may have been picked up during foreign vacations in eastern and southeastern Europe, though also in Austria. Whether all cases of TBE reported to the German Federal Health Office were correctly diagnosed is also open to doubt. Documentation of laboratory findings alone is also inappropriate, since in areas of endemic occurrence in particular contamination or inoculation titers are high, regardless of the clinical manifestation of the disease in the population. The prevalence of TBE (i.e. the frequency of all cases at a given time) in Germany was approximately 44 cases in 1990, approximately 120 cases in 1993, approximately 300 cases in 1994, and approximately 200 cases in 1995; the increase seen in 1994 was probably due to a mild winter (high tick survival rates) and warm summer (greater recreational activity among the population).

> Active and passive immunization has been very effective in bringing down the prevalence and incidence rates in the past.

For example, after the introduction of comprehensive inoculation against TBE in Austria, the annual incidence of the disease fell from 677 cases in 1982 to 109 in 1995, a decrease of roughly 90 %. In Bavaria too a fall in the incidence of TBE was observed between 1982 and 1992, as a result of increased inoculation against the disease.

Country	Incidence of TBE per 100 000 inhabitants (1995)
Germany	0.27
Sweden	3.4
Austria	6.0
Czech and Slovak Republic	24.6
Parts of European Russia and western Siberia	50-100

Table 3.4: Incidence of TBE in a number of selected countries

In eastern Europe there has been an increase in the number of cases of TBE, presumably because of changes in the socioeconomic conditions. The collapse of the old political systems and the associated discontinuation of large-scale agriculture also resulted in new natural foci for ticks on fallow land. In Latvia the number of cases of TBE rose from 152 in 1985 to 1344 in 1995; at the same time there was a shift in the incidence of the disease between different age groups: in 1995 there were 46 new cases per 100 000 inhabitants in the 50-59 age group, but far fewer in younger age groups, e.g. 10 new cases per 100 000 inhabitants in children. In Latvia the proportion of TBE sufferers who were unemployed rose from 28 % in 1990 to 67 % in 1996.

The risk of developing TBE is particularly high in eastern and southeastern Europe, as can be seen from a consideration of incidence data (☞ Table 3.4).

References

Altpeter E.S., Meier C. (1992). Epidemiologische Aspekte der neurologischen Komplikationen der Lyme-Borreliose in der Schweiz. Schweiz. Med. Wschr. 122: 22-26

Anda P., Rodriguez I., de la Loma A., Fernandez M. V., Lozano A. (1993). A serological survey and review of clinical Lyme borreliosis in Spain. C. I. D. 16: 310-319

Anderson J.F. (1991). Epizootiology of Lyme borreliosis. Scand. J. Infect. Dis. Suppl. 77: 23-34

Asbrink E., Hovmark A. (1993). Classification, Geographic Variations, and Epidemiology of Lyme Borreliosis. Clin. Dermatol. 11: 353-357

Ayford J.S., Rees D.H.D. (1994). Lyme Borreliosis. Plenum Press, New York: 89-93

Azulay R.D., Azulay-Abulafia L., Sodre C. T., Azulay M.M. (1991). Lyme Disease in Rio de Janeiro, Brazil. Int. J. Derm. 30 (8): 569-571

Berglund J., Eitrem R., Ornstein K., Lindberg A., Ringer A., Elmrud H., Carlsson M., Runehagen A., Svanborg C., Norrby R. (1995). An epidemiologic study of Lyme disease in southern Sweden. New Engl. J. Med. 333 (20): 1319-1327

Böhme M., Schwenecke S., Fuchs E., Wiebecke D., Karch H. (1992). Screening of Blood Donors and Recipients for *Borrelia burgdorferi* Antibodies: No Evidence of *B. burgdorferi* Infection Transmitted by Transfusion. Infusionstherapie 19: 204-207

Börner T. (1995). Arboviren. In: Prange, H.: Infektionskrankheiten des ZNS. Chapman & Hall Verlag, London. 61-74

Burek V., Misic-Mayerus L, Maretic T. (1992). Antibodies to *Borrelia burgdorferi* in various population groups in Croatia. Scand. J. Infect. Dis. 24 (5): 683-684

Carlberg H., Naito S. (1991). Lyme Borreliosis. J. Derm. 18: 125-142

Cimmino M. A., Fumarola D., Sambri V., Accardo S. (1992). The Epidemiology of Lyme Borreliosis in Italy. Microbiologica 15: 419-424

Dekonenko E.J., Steere A.C., Berardi V.P., Kravchuk L.N. (1988). Lyme Borreliosis in the Soviet Union: A Cooperative US-USSR Report. J. I. D. 158 (4): 748-753

Fahrer H., van der Linde S.M., Saubain M.J., Gern L., Zhioua E., Aeschlimann A. (1991). The Prevalence and Incidence of Clinical and Asymptomatic Lyme Borreliosis in a Population at Risk. J. I. D. 163: 305-310

Farrell G.M., Marth E.H. (1991). *Borrelia burgdorferi*: another cause of foodborne illness? Int. J. of Food Microbio. 14: 247-260

Fingerle V., Goodman J.L., Johnson R.C., Kurtti T.J., Munderloh U.G., Wilske B. (1997). Human Granulocytic Ehrlichiosis in Southern Germany: Increased Seroprevalence in High-Risk Groups. J. Clin. Microbiol. 35 (12): 3244-3247

Gern L., de Marval F., Aeschlimann A. (1991). Comparative Considerations on the Epidemiology of Lyme Borreliosis and Tick-borne encephalitis in Switzerland. F. Dusbábek and V. Bukva (Eds.): Modern Acarolgy 1: 249-254

Gniel D. (1998). Die FSME in Osteuropa, Apotheken Journal 4: 1-4

Grummet R., Wietthhölter H., Riehs I. et al. (1992). Frühsommer-Meningoencephalitis-Impfung. Indikation und kritische Beurteilung neurologischer Impfkomplikationen. Dtsch. Med. Wschr. 117: 112-116

Gustafson R. (1994). Epidemiological studies of Lyme borreliosis and Tick-borne encephalitis. Scand. J. Inf. Dis. Suppl. 92: 1-63

Gustafson R., Forsgren M., Gardulf A., Granström M., Svenungsson B. (1993). Clinical Manifestations and Antibody Prevalence of Lyme Borreliosis and Tick-borne Encephalitis in Sweden: A Study in Five Endemic Areas Close to Stockholm. Scand. J. Infect. Dis. 25 (5): 595-603

Gustafson R., Svenungsson B., Forsgren M., Gardul A., Granstroem M. (1992). Two-year survey of the incidence of Lyme borreliosis and Tick-borne encephalitis in a high-risk population in Sweden. Eur. J. Clin. Microbiol. Infect. Dis. 11 (10): 894-900

Hassler D., Zöller L., Haude M., Hufnagel H.D., Sonntag H.G. (1992). Lyme-Borreliose in einem europäischen Endemiegebiet. Dtsch. Med. Wschr. 117: 767-774

Horst H. (1991). Einheimische Zeckenborreliose (Lyme-Krankheit) bei Mensch und Tier. Erlangen: Perimed-Fachbuch-Verl.-Ges.

Jaenson T.G.T., Fish D., Ginsberg H.S., Gray J.S., Mather T.N., Piesman J. (1991). Methods for Control of Tick Vectors of Lyme Borreliosis. Scand. J. Infect. Dis.-Suppl. 77: 151-157

Kaiser R. (1995). Tick-borne encephalitis in southern Germany. Lancet 345: 463

Kaiser R., Kern A., Fressle R. et al. (1996). Zeckenvermittelte Erkrankungen in Baden-Württemberg. Münch. Med. Wschr. 138: 647-652

Kaiser R., Neumann-Haefelin D. (1996). FSME-Erkrankungen im Schwarzwald. Deutsches Ärzteblatt 93: 380-381

Korenberg E.I., Kryuchechnikov V.N., Kovalevsky Y.V. (1993). Advances in investigations of Lyme borreliosis in the territory of the former USSR. Europ. J. Epidem. 9 (1): 86-91

Kuiper H., de Jongh B.M., Nauta A.P., Houwleing H., Wiessing L.G., Moll van Charante A.W., Spanjaard L. (1991). Lyme borreliosis in Dutch forestry workers. J. Infect. 23: 279-286

Kunz Ch. (1992). Tick-borne encephalitis in Europe. Acta leidensia 60: 1-14

La Scola B., Roult D. (1997). Minireview: Laboratory Diagnosis of Rickettsiosis: Current Approaches to Diagnosis of Old and New Rickettsiel Diseases. J. Clin. Microbiol. 35 (11): 2715-2727

Magid D., Schwartz B., Graft M.S., Schwartz J.S. (1992). Prevention of Lyme Disease after Tick Bites. N. Engl. J. Med. 327 (8): 532-541

Mather T.N., Wilson M.L., Moore S.I., Ribeiro J.M.C., Spielman A. (1989): Comparing the Relative Potential of Rodents as Reservoirs of the Lyme Disease Spirochete (*Borrelia burgdorferi*). Am. J. Epidemiol. 130: 143-150

Mauch E., Vogel P., Kotnhuver H.H., Hähnel A. (1990). Klinische Wertigkeit von Antiköpertitern gegen *Borrelia burgdorferi* und Titerverläufe bei neurologischen Krankheitsbildern. Nervenarzt 61: 98-104

Mautner V.F., Gittermann M., Freitag V., Schneider E. (1990). Zur Epidemiologie der *Borrelia burgdorferi*-Infektion. Nervenarzt 61: 94-97

Mock D.E., Brillhart D.B., Upton S.J. (1992). Field Ecology of Lyme Disease in Kansas. Kansas Med.: 246-249

Motiejunas L., Bunikis J., Barbour A.G., Sadziene A. (1994). Lyme Borreliosis in Lithuania. Scand J. Infect Dis. 26: 149-155

Pierer K., Köck T., Freidl W., Stünzner D., Pierer G., Marth E., Lechner H., Möse J.R. (1993). Prevalence of Antibodies to *Borrelia burgdorferi* Flagellin in Styrian Blood Donors. Zbl. Bakt. 279: 239-243

Ruzic-Sablijic E., Strle F., Cimperman J. (1993). The Ixodes Ricinus Tick as a Vector of *Borrelia burgdorferi* in Slovenia. Eur. J. Epidemiol. 9 (4): 396-400

Sigal L.H., Curran A.S. (1991). Lyme Disease: A Multifocal Worldwide Epidemic. Annu. Rev. Publ. Health. 12: 85-109

Smith H.V., Gray J.S., Mckenzie G. (1991). A Lyme Borreliosis Human Serosurvey of Asymptomatic Adults in Ireland. Zbl. Bakt. 275: 382-389

Stanchi N.O., Balague L.J. (1993). Lyme Disease: antibodies against *Borrelia burgdorferi* in farm workers in Argentina. Rev. Saúde Pública 27 (4): 305-307

Steere A.C. (1993). Lyme Disease-1993. Bulletin on the Rheumatic Disease 42 (6): 4-7

Sticht-Groh M., Martin R., Schmidt-Wolf I. (1988). Antibody Titer Determinations against *Borrelia burgdorferi* in Blood Donors and in Two Different Groups of Patients. Ann. N. Y. Acad. Sci. 539: 497-499

Strle F., Stantic-Pavlinic M. (1996). Lyme disease in Europe. New Engl. J. Med. 334 (12):803

Süß J. (1995). Frühsommer-Meningoencephalitis in den neuen Bundesländern. Deutsches Ärzteblatt 92: 1069-1071

Pathogenesis and immune defense

4. Pathogenesis and immune defense

4.1. Lyme borreliosis

4.1.1. Pathogenesis

The pathogenesis of Lyme borreliosis, with all its clinical manifestations and courses, is not yet fully understood. The possible courses of *Borrelia* infections are shown in Fig. 4.1.

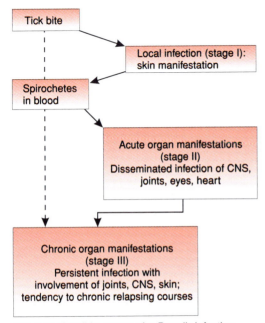

Fig. 4.1: Possible course of a *Borrelia* infection

First of all, a local infection develops at the puncture site; this infection may have skin manifestations and usually disappears spontaneously (☞ Section 5.1.2.1.). If spirochetes from the local infection site reach other organs via the blood, they can trigger symptoms there within a matter of weeks or months (acute organ manifestations). Months or even years after these symptoms have disappeared, fresh episodes of illness can occur (chronic organ manifestations). According to the usual division of Lyme borreliosis into disease stages,

- *Stage I* represents the stage of local infection
- *Stage II* corresponds to the acute organ manifestation (disseminated infection) and
- *Stage III* corresponds to the chronic organ manifestation (persistent infection)

For a case of Lyme borreliosis to be classified as stage III, progressive clinical symptoms must have been present for at least 6 months. (☞ Section 5.1.1.). However, the course of Lyme borreliosis described above, involving skin symptoms, early organ symptoms, and late organ symptoms, one after the other, is the exception rather than the rule. For example, organ manifestations may occur without the patient ever having noticed a local skin infection. Nor need there necessarily be a transition from acute to chronic organ manifestations. Finally, there have also been cases in which late manifestations have been diagnosed without any evidence of acute-stage symptoms in the patient's history.

4.1.1.1. Local infection

The *Borreliae* transmitted in the tick bite react with numerous host factors (☞ Fig. 4.2). *Borreliae* have been reported to be capable of attaching themselves to the cement substance of connective tissue (mucopolysaccharides) and to connective-tissue fibers (collagen). However, the effect of such interactions on the disease process cannot yet be conclusively established. It is also known that plasminogen binds to *Borreliae*, and can be activated to form plasmin on their surface. Plasmin (syn. fibrinolysin), a nonspecific endopeptidase, cleaves a large number of proteins. It is therefore conceivable that *Borrelia*-associated plasmin breaks down barriers (e.g. fibrin capsules and connective-tissue and vessel-wall structures), promoting spread of the pathogen. From this point on, the disease process is determined by the interaction between the spirochetes and local macrophages. The defense reactions begin with phagocytosis of the *Borreliae*. The phagocytosed bacteria are killed and fragments of the lysed pathogenic organisms presented to the immune system, allowing a specific immune response to the *Borreliae* to develop (☞ Section 4.1.2.). The interaction between *Borreliae* and macrophages also initiates a strong inflammatory reaction. The activated macrophages first secrete proinflammatory substances. These include monokines (TNFα, IL-1β, IL-6)

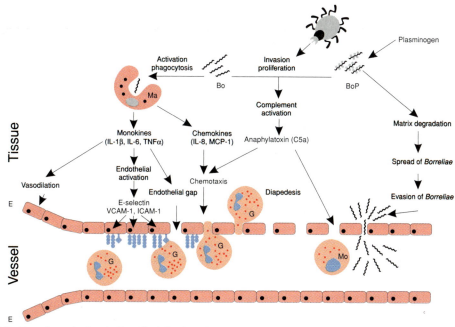

Fig. 4.2: Reactions in local *Borrelia* infection. **E**: Endothelial cells, **Ma**: Macrophage, **Mo**: Monocyte, **G**: Granulocyte, **Bo**: *Borreliae*, **BoP**: Plasmin-charged *Borreliae*

and chemokines (IL-8, MCP-1). The monokines trigger the expression of adhesion molecules (E-selectin, VCAM-1, ICAM-1) on endothelial cells. Vascular-system granulocytes increasingly adhere to these activated endothelial cells. At the same time the chemokines secreted by the macrophages induce emigration (diapedesis) of other granulocytes and monocytes from the vascular system and oriented migration (chemotaxis) of these cells to the site of infection. Since monokines increase vascular permeability, and blood flow is slowed down through the dilation of the vessels, nonspecific humoral defense factors (complement) reach the site of infection along with the granulocytes and monocytes. The complex inflammatory reaction may now be increased still further through *Borreliae* reacting with the complement system — either directly or indirectly through surface-associated plasmin — and producing the powerful inflammation mediator C5a with chemotactic and vasodilating action. In most cases of infection penetrating spirochetes are eliminated in the course of this inflammatory defense reaction. In a minority of cases, however, the nonspecific cellular and humoral defense factors that have accumulated in the area of inflammation are unable to terminate the disease process. As regards the progression of the disease, it is assumed that some *Borrelia* strains are strongly resistant to nonspecific defense mechanisms (☞ Section 4.1.2.).

4.1.1.2. Dissemination

The described vascular reactions in the area of inflammation allow *Borreliae* to slip in between the endothelial cells and out into the vascular lumen. Intracellular endothelial passage also seems to be possible. There are still no firm data on the subsequent course of infection (intravascular transport of the *Borreliae*, on the mechanism by which *Borreliae* evade from the vascular system, and on the reasons for the clinically conspicuous organotropism). Our current knowledge is limited to the observation that *B. afzelii* is more commonly the causative organism when there are skin manifestations and that *B. garinii* (OspA serotypes 4 and 6) is more common in infections of the CNS. It has been observed that plasmid loss causes *Borreliae* to lose their capacity for endothelial penetration, and this could indicate that plasmid-encoded factors are relevant to dissemination to frequently affected organs.

4.1.1.3. Acute organ manifestations

Manifest organ or tissue infection is accompanied by an inflammatory reaction. The underlying mechanisms are now only partly determined by interactions between *Borreliae* and nonspecific humoral and cellular defense factors (see above). Reactions of *Borreliae* with the products of the humoral defense system (antibodies and complement) and cellular defense system (activated T-lymphocytes; ☞ Section 4.1.2.) give rise to further inflammation mediators. The inflammatory reaction continues until specific and nonspecific defense mechanisms have eliminated the *Borreliae* (☞ Section 4.1.2. and Fig. 4. 3.).

4.1.1.4. Chronic organ manifestations

Less favorable clinical courses are observed mainly in those with chronic organ manifestations (☞ Section 5.1.1. and Section 7.1.2.). Some patients experience relapses alternating with symptom-free periods before lasting recovery. In other cases the disease enters a permanent chronic stage after repeated relapses. Cases of primary chronic courses are also known. This heterogeneity of Lyme borreliosis indicates that the immune defenses cannot always eliminate all the *Borreliae*. The persistence of *Borreliae* capable of reproduction obviously results in the establishment of an unstable state of equilibrium between the pathogen and the host. Each phase of disease activity is assumed to be accompanied by an increase in the number of pathogenic organisms, each increase setting in train fresh inflammatory reactions. The possible reasons for the survival of *Borreliae* in spite of the presence of a demonstrable immune response can at present only be guessed at (☞ Section 4.1.2.). An alternative reason for recurrent or chronic organ manifestations could lie in the persistence of inflammation-promoting constituents of *Borreliae* in tissue. Damaged *Borreliae* are known to develop blebs (membrane eversions) which contain mainly lipoproteins (OspA, OspB, OspC; ☞ Section 2.1.5.). These lipoproteins are powerful inductors of inflammatory reactions, as has been demonstrated for OspA. If such activators persist long enough, they can activate cells of the immune system nonspecifically (macrophages) and polyclonally (B- and T-lymphocytes) and initiate the release of inflammation mediators. Polyclonal activation of B-lymphocytes also carries the risk of a release of autoreactive antibodies that may in turn trigger inflammatory reactions in the affected organ (☞ Section 4.1.2.2.3.).

Spectrum of possible defense mechanisms	
Preimmune phase (= nonspecific defense before activation of the immune system)	**Immune phase** (= specific defense after activation of the immune system)
Phagocytosis of *Borreliae* by macrophages and intracellular destruction.	Increased phagocytosis after charging of *Borreliae* with phagocytosis-promoting ligands (IgG, C3b).
Inflammatory reaction mediated by monokines, chemokines, cytokines, and complement factors (extravasation of cellular (granulocytes, monocytes) and humoral defense factors (complement) from the vascular system and their concentration at the site of infection).	Intensified inflammatory reaction by increased release of monokines, chemokines, interleukins, and complement factors.
Destruction of *Borreliae* by complement after antibody-independent classical activation (no action on B. afzelii strains).	Increased destruction of *Borreliae* by complement after classical activation in the presence of antibodies (but patient sera differ strongly in their content of *Borrelia*-destroying protective antibodies).
Extracellular destruction of *Borreliae* by release of toxic factors from phagocytes (hypothetical).	Extracellular destruction of *Borreliae* by release of toxic factors from phagocytes (hypothetical).
	Immobilization of mobile *Borreliae* by antibodies, hence inhibition of local spread of the pathogen and vascular invasion and evasion (hypothetical).

Fig. 4.3: Spectrum of possible defense mechanisms

4.1.2. Immune defense

The *Borrelia*-infected organism has numerous defense strategies for preventing the development of disease. The body combats the disease so successfully that only a small number of people infected with *Borreliae* actually develop symptoms, which is to say that most cases of Lyme borreliosis clear up spontaneously, without antibiotic therapy (☞ Section 5.1.1.). As the duration of infection increases, the range of defense mechanisms becomes even wider (☞ Fig. 4.3).

In the early phase of infection, only nonspecific defenses are available to combat the pathogen. This is the preimmune phase. Once the immune response has been triggered, the arsenal of defense mechanisms is supplemented by the specific reaction products of the immune system (immune phase).

4.1.2.1. Preimmune phase

In the preimmune phase (☞ Fig. 4.3) *Borreliae* transmitted by tick bites are confronted with nonspecific defense cells (macrophages, granulocytes) at the site of the local infection, the number of such cells increasing as the inflammatory reaction becomes more intense (☞ Section 4.1.1 and Fig. 4.2). At this stage *Borreliae* are already phagocytosed and destroyed intracellularly. *Borreliae* are also exposed to the complement system. This system helps the body to defend itself by speeding up the phagocytosis of *Borreliae* (C3b opsonization) or killing bacteria directly (C5b-9 membrane attack complex). However, *Borrelia* strains differ in their capacity to activate the complement system in the presence of antibodies. Strains of the genospecies *B. afzelii* in particular are resistant to the complement system — they prevent the membrane attack complex from forming on their surface. This resistance mechanism could thus give some *Borrelia* strains a better chance of local survival and so contribute to the development of a manifest infection.

4.1.2.2. Immune phase

Once infection has taken place, the immune phase (☞ Fig. 4.3) begins, in which the antibodies are formed. However, antibodies are not detectable until 2 to 3 weeks after infection at the earliest (☞ Section 6.1.3.2.1.). Immunoglobulins of classes IgM and IgG activate the complement system, strengthening the phagocytosis (C3b opsonization) and complement-mediated destruction (C5b-9 membrane attack complex) of *Borreliae*. However, studies of the *Borrelia*-destroying effect of patient sera have shown that not all sera can kill *Borreliae*, despite the presence of antibodies. It can therefore be concluded that only antibodies with a certain (as yet unknown) specificity have a protective effect and that not every infected person produces these antibodies.

Here we see a possible gap in the defenses of the specific immune defense system, and one that could have adverse consequences particularly in respect of *B. afzelii* strains, which are highly resistant to complement. Despite recognizable weaknesses, a **strong** humoral **immune defense system** is of decisive importance for a successful control of a *Borrelia* infection (☞ Fig. 4.4). In contrast, the contribution of the cellular immune defense system to the elimination of *Borreliae* is small. In a few isolated cases strengthened cellular immune defenses actually seem to have an adverse effect on the disease process (☞ Section 4.1.2.2.3.).

4.1.2.2.1. Reinfections

The immune response to a *Borrelia* infection can provide long-lasting immunity. One obvious explanation for this is that antibodies remain detectable for years and are thus able to exert their protective effects over a long time. However, there are also unequivocal cases of reinfection. There are many reasons for this. A second infection can occur in cases where the **immune response is weak** as a result of very early antibiotic therapy following a tick bite in the past (☞ Fig. 4.4, item 2). Another possible explanation for reinfections is that protective antibodies account for only a small part of the humoral immune response, and that after reaching a peak they disappear again within weeks or months. **Waning immunity**, with a risk of another infection, would be the result (☞ Fig. 4.4, item 3). There could also be a risk of a reinfection if the initial infection did not lead to an **appropriate immune response** (☞ Fig. 4.4, item 4). Such a situation would occur if the reinfection involved a *Borrelia* strain with an antigen profile different from that of the strain responsible for the initial infection. Sufficient cross-immunity would not be guaranteed in such cases. Unfortunately, current

4.1.2.2.2. Persistence of *Borreliae*

Borreliae can survive in infected persons despite all efforts of the humoral immune defense system, resulting in relapses, late manifestations, and chronic courses, though overall these constitute only a small fraction of the possible courses (☞ Section 5.1.1.). There is as yet no satisfactory explanation for the persistence of the pathogens. What could be happening is that in infections with *Borrelia* the onset of antibody formation is unusually slow and the quantities of protective antibodies formed too small, reducing the effectiveness of the humoral immune defense system (☞ Fig. 4.4, item 2). In such situations it is conceivable that the *Borreliae* make use of the prolonged preimmune phase to withdraw to regions where they are protected from the slowly forming antibodies. No such protective niches are yet known, but they may be located both extracellularly and intracellularly (endothelial cells, fibroblasts) in the CNS, locomotor apparatus, or other preferred sites of infection. Survival of *Borreliae* in spite of a demonstrable humoral response may be also be promoted by their ability to change their antigens. There is evidence that after longer periods of culture *Borrelia* antigens are in some instances no longer expressed (☞ Section 2.1.4.). Antibodies produced in response to these antigens would thus no longer have any protective function, so **an immune response that is no longer appropriate** could be the reason for pathogen persistence in such instances. (☞ Fig. 4.4, item 5). A particularly unfavorable situation promoting the persistence of *Borreliae* thus arises from the combined occurrence of various factors:

- 1. Infection with a *Borrelia* strain having a high degree of complement resistance
- 2. Escape of *Borreliae* to a niche where they are protected from the immune defense system
- 3. Unusually weak humoral immune response
- 4. Lack of protective antibodies, with restricted antibody spectrum
- 5. An immune response that is no longer appropriate, following a change of the antigen by the *Borreliae* (mimicry)

4.1.2.3. Immunopathology

The protective humoral immune response is associated with preferential formation of TH2-lymphocytes, which in turn stimulate the B-lymphocytes to form antibodies. The regulation of the humoral immune response, including B-lymphocyte maturation and antibody secretion, is affected by interleukins, among which IL-4 plays a decisive role. Stimulation of a cellular immune re-

\multicolumn{2}{c}{Interactions between immune response and course of infection (hypothetical)}	
1. Immune response *strong*: Course of infection:	Quick and intense formation of protective antibodies (IgM and IgG) and efficient destruction of *Borreliae*. Spontaneous recovery in localized and early disseminated infections; risk of *Borrelia* persistence low.
2. Immune response *weak*: Course of infection:	Delayed and weak formation of antibodies (only IgM, little IgM and IgG), small amounts of protective antibodies. Localized disease, early or late organ manifestations, risk of persistence of *Borreliae* with relapses and chronic illness elevated.
3. Immune response *declining*: Course of infection:	Falling antibody levels after the illness, with loss of immunity. Relapses with persistence of *Borreliae* after the first infection, danger of reinfection.
4. Immune response *not appropriate*: Course of infection:	Good antibody levels after the infection but with pronounced species- or serotype-specificity of the antibodies formed, the immunity is restricted to the pathogen and closely related strains of *Borrelia*. Risk of a reinfection with a *Borrelia* strain having a different set of antigens.
5. Immune response *no longer appropriate*: Course of infection:	Good and persistent antibody levels after the infection, loss of antibody reactivity against the pathogen following a change in the antigen pattern of the *Borrelia* strain. Risk of persistence of *Borreliae* with a tendency toward relapses.
6. Immune response *pathological*: Course of infection:	Strong TH1 immune reaction with release of inflammatory cytokines by activated T lymphocytes and activated macrophages, TH2 immune response (antibody formation) rather weak, autoreactive antibodies through polyclonal activation of B lymphocytes? Tendency toward relapses and chronic courses with very strong inflammatory reactions.

Fig. 4.4: Interactions between the immune response and the course of infection (hypothetical)

sponse with the formation of inflammatory TH1-cells which activate macrophages via secreted INF-γ does not seem to be necessary for combating Borrelia infections. Recent observations even suggest that in Lyme borreliosis patients with particularly strong inflammatory activity the underlying cause could be a **pathological immune response** with preferential TH1-activation (☞ Fig. 4.4, item 6). Increased levels of IL-12, which has a positive influence on the cellular immune response, have been detected in the inflammation regions affected (e.g. joint puncture fluid), lending support to such ideas. The pathogenetic significance of immune-response dysregulation would be even greater if there were not only an increase in TH1-activation but also a simultaneous decrease in activation of TH2. Very strong inflammatory reactions would be expected in such patients, with recurrent and chronic courses of the disease. So far, however, a definitive assessment of the true significance of immune response dysregulation with preferential TH1-activation for the pathogenesis of Lyme borreliosis cannot be carried out. The possible formation of autoreactive antibodies after polyclonal activation of B-lymphocytes has already been referred to above (☞ Section 4.1.1.4.), but it is not clear at present whether autoimmune reactions play any role in the pathogenesis of Lyme borreliosis (☞ Fig. 4.4, item 6).

4.2. Tick-borne encephalitis (TBE)

4.2.1. Pathogenesis

The TBE virus is transmitted to humans through the bite of a virus-infected tick.

The viruses first multiply locally in the skin cells (☞ Fig. 4.5) and subsequently find their way to regional lymph nodes via the draining lymph vessels, and from there into the bloodstream via the large lymph tracts. Various tissue and organ cells are infected in the primary viremia phase that now follows (connective tissue, smooth muscle, skeletal muscle, myocardium, exocrine and endocrine glands, monocytic phagocyte system). In a progressive infection a second viremic phase then develops, in which the TBE virus invades the central nervous system. The brain presumably becomes infected after viral multiplication in endothelial cells of the cerebral capillaries. In the infected brain the viruses spread from cell to cell, affecting both neurons and neuroglial cells. The infection leads not only to direct damage to the cells of the central nervous system, but also triggers opposing reactions by the body (build-up of lymphocytes, plasma cells, macrophages, and neuroglial cells; interstitial cerebral edema). Meningeal exudation can also occur in defense reactions. In severe courses the neuronal damage is so pronounced that full recovery is no longer possible. In particularly severe cases the disease can even prove fatal (☞ Section 5.2. and Fig. 5.11).

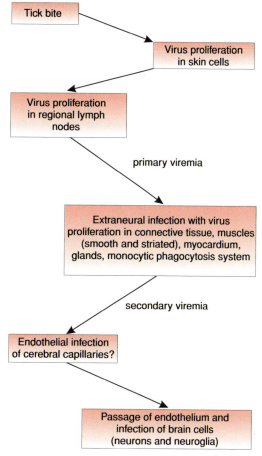

Fig. 4.5: Possible course of an TBE virus infection

4.2.2. Immune defense

The second viremic phase, in which the central nervous system is infected, occurs in only about 35 % of the patients, in whom extraneural tissue and organ infection with the TBE virus has occurred (☞ above and Fig. 4.5). It seems that in most patients further hematogenic spread of the virus is effectively prevented by the defense reactions of the immune system. The immune defenses are directed against the virus-infected cells, which are recognized and destroyed by cytotoxic T-lymphocytes. Antibodies may also play a role in the lysis of virus-infected cells, by binding to infection-induced non-viral antigens (glycoprotein NS1) and initiating cell destruction with the aid of the complement. The body combats further intracellular virus multiplication with these lytic defense mechanisms, but the immune defenses are also directed against the virus itself. The main protection comes from antibodies to coat protein E (☞ Section 2.2.3.). Reaction with these antibodies neutralizes the TBE viruses, i.e. they lose their capacity to adsorb onto cells and to infect them. Lysis of virus-infected cells and virus neutralization mean that in most cases the disease is terminated at the extraneural infection stage. The conditions for an infection of the brain only occur where a particularly massive extraneural multiplication of the virus has occurred and the immune response is not sufficient to prevent hematogenic infection of the central nervous system.

References

Breitner-Ruddock S., Würzner R., Schulze J., Brade V. (1997). Heterogeneity in the complement-dependent bacteriolysis within the species of *Borrelia burgdorferi*. Med. Microbiol. Immunol. 185: 253-260

Cinco M., Murgia R., Presani G., Perticarari S. (1997). Integrin CR3 mediates the binding of nonspecifically opsonized *Borrelia burgdorferi* to human phagocytes and mammalian cells. Infect. Immun. 65: 4784-4789

Coleman J.L., Sellati T.J., Testa J.E., Kew R.R., Furie M.B., Benach J.L. (1995). *Borrelia burgdorferi* binds plasminogen, resulting in enhanced penetration of endothelial monolayers. Infect Immun 63: 2478-2484

Fuchs H., Wallich R., Simon M.M., Kramer M.D. (1994). The outer surface protein A of the spirochete *Borrelia burgdorferi* is a plasmin(ogen) receptor. Proc. Natl. Acad. Sci. USA 91: 12594-12598

Guo B.P., Norris S.J., Rosenberg L.C., Höök M. (1995). Adherence of *Borrelia burgdorferi* to the Proteoglycan Decorin. Infect. Immun. 63: 3467-3472

Hu L.T., Klempner M.S. (1997). Host-pathogen interactions in the immunopathogenesis of Lyme disease. J. Clin. Immunol.17: 354-365

Infante-Duarte C., Kamradt T. (1997). Lipopeptides of *Borrelia burgdorferi* outer surface proteins induce Th1 phenotype development in $\alpha\beta$ T-cell receptor transgenic mice. Infect. Immun. 65: 4094-4099

Kraiczy P., Peters S., Seitz C., Würzner R., Oschmann P., Brade V. (1998). Growth inhibitory and bactericidal efficacy of sera from Lyme borreliosis patients on *B. burgdorferi* strains. Wien. Klin. Wochschr. 110: 886-893

Kramer M.D., Wallich R., Simon M.M. (1996). The outer surface protein A (OspA) of *Borrelia burgdorferi*: A vaccine candidate and bioactive mediator. Infection 24: 190-194

Matyniak J.E., Reiner S.L. (1995). T helper phenotype and genetic susceptibility in experimental Lyme disease. J. Exp. Med. 181: 1251-1254

Monath T.P., Heinz F.X. (1996) Flaviviruses. In: Virology, Fields B.N., Knipe D.M., Howley P.M. (Eds.) Lippincott - Raven Publishers, Philadelphia: 961-1034

Oksi J., Savolainen J., Pene J., Bousquet J., Laippala P., Viljanen M.K. (1996). Decreased interleukin-4 and increased gamma interferon production by peripheral blood mononuclear cells of patients with Lyme borreliosis. Infect Immun 64: 3620-3623

Padilla M.L., Callister S.M., Schell R.F., Bryant G.L., Jobe D.A., Lovrich S.D., DuChateau B.K., Jensen J.R. (1996). Characterization of the protective borreliacidal antibody response in humans and hamsters after vaccination with *Borrelia burgdorferi* outer surface protein A vaccine. J. Infect. Dis. 174: 739-746

Pavia C.S., Wormser G.P., Norman G.L. (1997). Activity of sera from patients with Lyme disease against *Borrelia burgdorferi*. Clin. Infect. Dis. 25 (1): 25-30

Philipp M.T., Johnson B.J.B. (1994). Animal models of Lyme disease: pathognesis and immunoprophylaxis. Trends Microbiol. 2: 431-437

Piesman J., Dolan M.C., Happ C.M., Luft B.J., Rooney S.E., Mather T.N., Golde W.T. (1997). Duration of immunity to reinfection with tick-transmitted *Borrelia burgdorferi* in naturally infected mice. Infect. Immun. 65: 4043-4047

Seiler K.P., Weis J.J. (1996). Immunity to Lyme disease: protection, pathology and persistence. Curr. Opin. Immunol. 8: 503-509

Sellati T.J., Abrescia L.D., Radolf J.D., Furie M.B. (1996). Outer surface lipoproteins of *Borrelia burgdorferi* activate vascular endothelium in vitro. Infect. Immun. 64: 3180-3187

Sigal L.H. (1997). Lyme Disease: A review of aspects of its immunology and immunopathogenesis. Annu. Rev. Immunol. 65:63-92

Sprenger H., Krause A., Kaufmann A., Priem S., Fabian D., Burmester G.R., Gemsa D., Rittig M.G. (1997). *Borrelia burgdorferi* induces chemokines in human monocytes. Infect. Immun. 65: 4384-4388

Van Dam A.P., Oei A., Jaspars R., Fijen C., Wilske B., Spanjaard L., Dankert J. (1997). Complement-mediated serum sensitivity among spirochetes that cause Lyme disease. Infect. Immun. 65: 1228-1236

Clinical symptoms

5. Clinical symptoms

5.1. Lyme borreliosis

5.1.1. Course of infection and stages

Lyme borreliosis is a multisystem disease which develops in stages (☞ Table 5.1). It involves mainly the skin, joints, and the nervous system. It is classified into stages on a clinical basis, according to the time of infection or, if the patient is unaware of having suffered a tick bite, the duration of illness. The disease can

- pass through all three stages one after the other
- jump a stage or
- first manifest itself in any of the stages.

According to the results of animal studies the incidence of infection after a bite by an infected tick is 7 % (36 h) to 75 % (48 h), depending on how long it had fed. In about 5 % of the cases (manifestation rate) clinical symptoms occur, affecting mainly the skin. Spontaneous recovery, sometimes in association with seroconversion, occurs in the remaining cases (☞ Fig. 5.1).

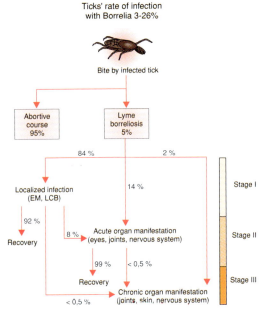

Fig. 5.1: Course of infection in European Lyme borreliosis (some of the percentages given are projections obtained by combining data from a number of European epidemiological studies with our own)

Stage I (localized infection)	Stage II (acute organ manifestation)	Stage III (chronic organ manifestation)

• Dermatoborreliosis
  - Erythema migrans
  - Lymphadenosis cutis benigna
• Nonspecific symptoms (myalgias, arthralgias, fever)
	• Neuroborreliosis
	  - Meningitis
	  - Meningoradicul(oneur)itis
	  - Meningoradicul(omyel)(oencephal)itis
	  - Cerebrovascular course form
	  - Myositis
	• Internistic manifestations
	  - Mono(oligo)arthritis
	  - Endo(myo)(peri)carditis
	  - Hepatitis
	• Ophthalmoborreliosis
	  - Chorioretinitis
	  - Inflammation of optic nerves
	  - Uveitis
		• Neuroborreliosis
		  - ACA-associated mono-(poly)neuritis
		  - Progressive encephalomyelitis
		  - Cerebrovascular course form
		• Dermatoborreliosis
		  - Acrodermatitis chronica atrophicans
		  - Lymphadenosis cutis benigna
		  - Circumscribed scleroderma (?)
		• Mono(poly)arthritis

Table 5.1: Stages and syndromes involved in Lyme borreliosis

Stage I

The disease usually begins after a 5- to 48-day incubation period (median interval 12 days), with the appearance of erythema migrans at the site of the tick bite. About 20 % of patients complain of influenza-like symptoms with muscle and joint pains, symptoms of the hematogenic dissemination which has already occurred. Studies in the USA have given markedly higher percentages, 70 to 80 %. Lymphadenosis cutis benigna and multiple erythemata migrantia are rarely described as the leading symptom. The liver and kidney laboratory values may be increased. Without antibiotic treatment spontaneous recovery from stage I infection without sequelae occurs in over 90 % of the cases.

Stage II

The second stage of the disease begins 2-10 weeks after infection. In half of the cases the clinical course is biphasic. Spontaneous healing of the erythema is followed by secondary symptoms of organ manifestations

- in the peripheral nervous system
- in the meninges
- in joints
- in the heart
- in the eyes.

In 80 % of the cases the erythema migrans is already gone at the time of the first consultation with the doctor. One sufferer in seven remains asymptomatic throughout stage I, and primary hematogenic or lymphogenic colonization of the organs occurs with the occurrence of acute symptoms. The principal clinical sign at this stage of the disease is lymphocytic meningoradiculitis (Bannwarth's syndrome). Without treatment, weeks or months of illness are followed by spontaneous remission in 99 % of the cases, with only partial recovery in one-third of the cases.

Stage III

In contrast to the often self-limiting course of stages I and II, tertiary Lyme borreliosis is characterized by a chronic, inflammatory, organ-destroying disease process in the skin, joints, or the nervous system. The progressive disease must, by definition, have been present for more than 6 months if it is to be classified as stage III. This period was chosen because it can be shown on the basis of the spontaneous course in untreated cases that complete recovery can no longer be expected unless remission has already started by this time. The incubation time is not known with certainty. In cases of tertiary neuroborreliosis with clinically documented erythema migrans (EM) the interval between EM and the onset of neurological symptoms was 4-12 months. Data in the literature giving latency periods of 1.5 to 17 years for neuroborreliosis are questionable, as they are usually based on reports of a tick bite in the medical history. Latency periods of several years have been reported in patients with acrodermatitis chronica atrophicans preceded by erythema migrans. In the majority of cases the disease follows a primary chronic-progressive course. In the remaining cases stage I or II of the disease was present earlier, so the disease follows a secondary chronic-progressive course. Case reports in which patients had passed through all three stages are very rare. Spontaneous remissions of tertiary Lyme borreliosis have never been described.

5.1.2. Organ manifestations and the associated syndromes

The relative frequency of the different organ manifestations varies according to the size of the study, the diagnostic criteria, and the geographic region studied.

- Erythema migrans: *65-75 %*
- Lymphadenosis cutis benigna: *1-3 %*
- Acrodermatitis chronica atrophicans: *1-2 %*
- Neuroborreliosis: *10-12 %*
- Lyme arthritis: *8 %* (Europe), *30 %* (USA)
- Carditis: *0.2-3 %*
- Ophthalmoborreliosis: *0.2 %*

Essentially, Lyme arthritis seems to be substantially more common in the USA, while neuroborreliosis and ACA occur more often in Europe. Genotype-specific differences in organotropism between *B. burgdorferi* s.s. and *Borrelia garinii* or *afzelii* may play a role in this respect (☞ Sections 2.1.5. and 4.1.1.2.).

5.1.2.1. Dermatoborreliosis

5.1.2.1.1. Erythema (chronicum) migrans (E[C]M) — stage I

The most common cuteneous manifestation is erythema migrans (☞ Fig. 5.2a-d), which can only be described as chronic if it lasts more than 4 weeks.

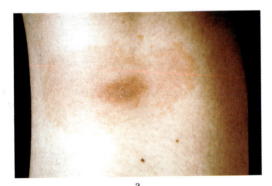

a

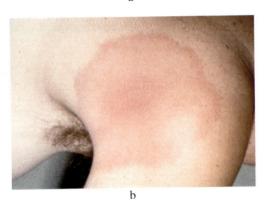

b

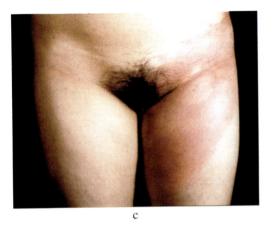

c

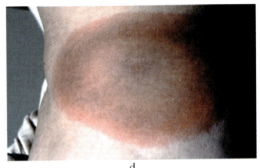

d

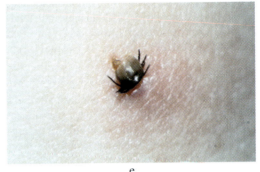

e

Fig. 5.2a-e: Erythema (chronicum) migrans and insect-bite reaction. **a-d:** The figures show a number of variants of EM. **e**: Insect bite reaction. The figure shows an acute skin reaction following a tick bite. (With the kind permission of Prof. Schill and Dr. Niemeier, Giessen University Dermatological Clinic)

It can occur from a few days to several weeks after a bite by a tick (rarely by another insect), whatever the age of the patient, but only about 40 % of such patients can remember having been bitten by a tick.

> The efflorescence has a sharp boundary with a central lymphocytic nodule and a pronounced halo. It spreads rapidly over the course of a few days, and the erythema fades slowly from the center outward. An extensive area of livid reddening and swelling is occasionally observed.

Atypical variants such as irregular blotchy, flaky, or hemorrhagic erythema are sometimes observed. If left untreated, the EM disappears within on average 28 days. Persistence for several months or up to a year is very rare. Multiple erythemas as an expression of hematogenic dissemination are substantially less common in Europe than in the USA, occurring in about 5 % compared with about 48 % of the patients. Half of the patients affected report painful dysesthesias with numb areas as an expression of local cutaneous neuritis in the region covered by the efflorescence. Clinical signs of general infection are present in 20 % of the cases.

> The observation that patients with pronounced concomitant symptoms are more often among those who develop stage II is prognostically important.

 Differential diagnosis

In differential diagnostics it is necessary to consider the following possibilities in addition to a common insect-bite reaction:

- streptogenic erysipelas
- allergic drug exanthem
- exanthema anulare centrifugale, and
- tinea corporis.

In order to distinguish insect bite reactions, European experts have agreed to a minimum exanthem diameter of 5 cm. **Histopathologically**, interstitial and perivascular lymphocytic cell infiltrates can be detected in the middle and deep layers of the dermis. Endothelial swellings, fibrin deposits, and erythrocyte extravasates, as signs of vasculitis, regularly occur around the edges of the erythema.

5.1.2.1.2. Lymphadenosis cutis benigna (LCB) — stage I/III

A massive lymphocytic reaction may lead to the development of a *Borrelia* lymphocytoma known as lymphadenosis cutis benigna (☞ Fig. 5.3a).

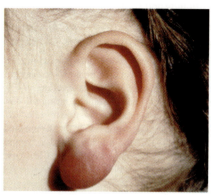
a

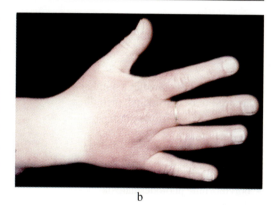
b

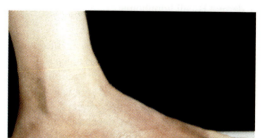
c

Fig. 5.3a-c: **a**: Lymphadenosis cutis benigna. **b**: Acrodermatitis chronica atrophicans, inflammatory edematous phase. **c**: Acrodermatitis chronica atrophicans, final atrophic stage. (With the kind permission of Prof. Schill and Dr. Niemeier, Giessen University Dermatological Clinic.)

This can occur in the course of acrodermatitis chronica atrophicans, either in stage I or in stage III.

> Lymphadenosis cutis benigna comprises a livid red puffy swelling or nodule due to lymphoreticular cell proliferation in the cutis and/or subcutis. *Borrelia* lymphocytomas are common in areas of soft and well-perfused tissue such as the earlobes and nipples. They may be between 0.5 and 5 cm in diameter.

If left untreated, LCB can persist for several months or even up to a year. The *Borrelia* lymphocytoma can occur at the same time as erythema migrans, it can follow it, or it can develop far from the primary point of entry. In cases of acrodermatitis chronica atrophicans (ACA) a lymphocytoma can develop inside or outside the affected skin area.

Differential diagnosis

In **differential diagnostics** a number of skin reactions need to be considered, including:
- insect bite reactions
- histiocytoma
- sarcoidosis
- granuloma eosinophilicum faciei
- polymorphic photodermatosis
- pseudolymphomatoid drug reactions
- dermal B-cell lymphoma
- lupus erythematodus

Histology can considerably assist differential diagnostics. In characteristic cases it is possible to detect lymphoradicular cell proliferations which develop into a lymph-node like structure with approximately rounded reaction centers. Large or small germinal centers may develop (centroblasts and centrocytes), with lymphocytes and germinal center macrophages. These are often accompanied by plasma cells and occasionally by eosinophilic granulocytes. As in ACA, destruction of the elastic tissue and atrophy of the cutaneous appendages can be detectable.

5.1.2.1.3. Acrodermatitis chronica atrophicans (ACA) — stage III

This clinical picture (☞ Fig. 5.3b+c) is regarded as the typical stage III manifestation of Lyme borreliosis and is observed in 1 to 2 % of all patients. It is difficult to determine the mean incubation time of ACA, as the condition develops slowly and the onset can be difficult to pinpoint with any accuracy. ACA can develop from erythema migrans, and latency periods of 6 months to 3 years have been described in such cases. The condition affects mainly older patients and women. In adolescents ACA is rare. The condition generally starts out with patches of erythema or livid red swellings positioned asymmetrically on the extensor surfaces of the extremities (inflammatory edematous phase) and progresses into the final atrophic stage over a period of years or decades. Clinically, there is an increasing atrophy of the dermal and epidermal tissue, with thinning of the epidermis until it becomes like cigarette paper coupled with increased projection of the underlying blood vessels. Striated areas of redness and funicles can develop on the extensor surfaces of the lower arm, and in rare cases the lower leg, taking the form of ulnar stripes (in approximately 25 %) or tibial stripes (in approx. 4 %). Excessive formation of new connective tissue leads to the development of hard, ivory-colored, dermatosclerotic plates with armor-like thickening of the skin close to the joints in about 16 % of the cases and often (some 25 %) to juxta-articular fibrinoid nodules. If it persists for a fairly long time, the ACA can spread to the contralateral extremity. All four limbs are sometimes affected. The consequences of the local inflammatory process may include symptoms of disease in the skeleton (30 %) and nervous system (40 %). ACA-associated polyneuritis, focal nodular myositis, and destructive arthritis with bone alterations (atrophy, thickening of the cortex) have been described in such cases.

Differential diagnosis

In **differential diagnostics** the possibility of congestive dermatitis with chronic venous insufficiency or acrocyanosis should be considered. Typically, the early edematous stage is characterized **histopathologically** by edema in the dermis and dilation of blood and lymph vessels. Perivascular lymphoplasmacytic infiltrates can be observed. Atrophic changes affecting the elastic tissue in the region of the inflammatory infiltrate can be apparent early on. The collagen fibers swell up and become homogeneous. The atrophy also affects the subcutaneous fatty tissue and the sebaceous glands and follicles.

■ Case history — ACA-associated polyneuritis with arthritis — stage III

A 75-year-old woman reported increasingly severe burning sensation in both feet for 8 months, increasing uncertainty of gait, and for 4 months swelling and hyperthermia of the left knee and ankle during the day. The clinical and neurological examination revealed the typical finding for the edematous stage of ACA in the lower left leg, swelling of the left knee, and a symmetrical mainly sensory polyneuropathy. The Achilles tendon reflexes were absent on both sides. There was a sock-shaped area of hypoesthesia and hypoalgesia, reaching to below the knee. The serum laboratory values were normal, apart from an accelerated ESR of 40/65 mm after Westergren. The cerebrospinal fluid values were in the normal range. Both the ELISA for *Borrelia* and the immunoblot showed pronounced IgG immunoreactivity

5.1. Lyme borreliosis

in the serum. Only low concentrations of IgM antibodies were detected. Both the oligoarthritis and the ACA were cured without sequelae by 3 weeks of treatment with 1 × 2 g/day of ceftriaxone. Weakened ATRs and a diminished sensitivity to vibrations remained as residual damage caused by the ACA-associated polyneuritis. The IgG antibody concentrations had fallen slightly after one year. IgM antibodies were no longer detectable.

5.1.2.1.4. Circumscribed scleroderma, lichen sclerosis et atrophicus (stage III)

There is some evidence of an etiopathogenetic association between Lyme borreliosis and circumscribed scleroderma (morphea). It has been suggested that the cases described should be interpreted as pseudoscleroderma within the context of ACA. The distinctly increased incidence of *B. burgdorferi*-specific antibodies in a large group of patients (n = 210) with circumscribed scleroderma (31 %) compared with a control group (4 %) supports an association. Spirochete-like organisms have also been isolated by culture and histologically from skin specimens obtained from scleroderma foci. In some cases antibiotics have been used successfully.

Lichen sclerosus et atrophicus is another dermatosis which is histomorphologically similar to both ACA and circumscribed scleroderma. Once again there have been repeated references to a possible association, so far without definitive proof.

5.1.2.2. Neuroborreliosis

Neuroborreliosis occurs in about 10 to 12 % of patients with Lyme borreliosis. The incidence in Germany is 5.8 to 10 per 100 000 and in Sweden up to 0.6 to 2.4 per 100 000. Typically, it develops during stage II and III of the disease. The occurrence of this organ manifestation in stage I is disputed. It is not uncommon for patients in the early stages of the disease to complain of headaches. If the cerebrospinal fluid shows signs of inflammation in these patients then, according to our definition, the patient should be assigned to stage II (acute organ manifestations). The situation is different when patients have painful paresthesias in the region of the EM. This could be regarded as a clinical correlate of cutaneous neuritis, and could thus be assigned to the stage of localized infection.

B. burgdorferi can infect the entire neural axis and lead to a wide spectrum of neurological manifestations:

- mono(poly)neuritis
- lymphocytic meningitis
- myositis
- chorioretinitis
- meningoradiculitis
- paraplegic myelitis
- myeloradiculitis
- focal or generalized encephalitis with
  - extrapyramidal motor symptoms
  - cerebellar ataxia
  - hemiparesis
  - exogenous psychosis
  - epileptic attacks
- cerebral vasculitis with cerebral infarction and
- progressive encephalomyelitis.

All these syndromes may be observed alone or in combination. Monosymptomatic courses are rare, at 8 %.

Most patients with neuroborreliosis become ill between June and October (☞ Fig. 5.4). Up to 40 % of patients remember having had a tick bite. All age groups can be affected (☞ Fig. 5.5).

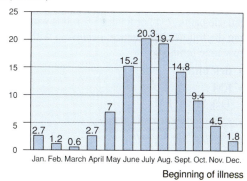

Fig. 5.4: Seasonal pattern of the onset of illness, based on 330 patients with neuroborreliosis

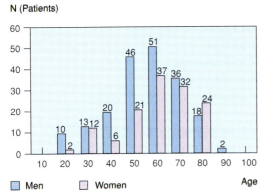

Fig. 5.5: Age and sex distribution in 330 adult patients with neuroborreliosis

After an incubation period of a few days to weeks, 32 to 49 % of those who later suffer neuroborreliosis after a tick bite notice erythema migrans. This is the first sign of illness in 96 % of the cases. Another common leading syndrome is radicular or pseudoradicular pain, which is reported by 70 % of patients with neuroborreliosis (☞ Table 5.2).

The radicular or pseudoradicular pains are present at the onset of the disease in 41 % of the patients. In rare cases neuroborreliosis starts out with paresis of the cranial nerves (12 %), headaches (10 %), muscle pains (7 %) or fever (5 %). It is worth noting the following sequence, occurring within narrow time limits:

- **tick bite**
- **EM**
  Tick bite to EM:
  - *median interval* 12 days
  - *range* 5 to 48 days
- **radicular pain**
  EM to pain:
  - *median interval* 8 days
  - *range* 0 to 95 days

and finally

- **neurological deficit**
  EM to deficit:
  - *median interval* 40 days
  - *range* 0 to 150 days.

Finding	Incidence
Tick bite	37 %
Erythema (chronicum) migrans	34 %
Radicular pain	70 %
Headaches	18 %
Muscle pains	13 %
Fever	10 %
Arthralgias	1.5 %
Arthritis	3 %
Carditis	1 %
Acrodermatitis chronica atrophicans	1.5 %
Chorioretinitis	0.3 %
Hepatitis (chemical laboratory findings)	42 %
Myositis	0.3 %
Paresis	
- peripheral	45 %
- central	9 %
Sensory disorders	
- peripheral	44 %
- central	4 %
Involvement of cranial nerves	
- n. facialis	39 %
- other	8 %
Bladder disturbances	5 %
Organic psychosyndrome	3 %
Cerebellar ataxia	2 %
Parkinson's disease	1.2 %
Stroke	1.2 %

Table 5.2: Symptoms and findings in neuroborreliosis (n = 330; multiple answers could be given)

Almost 60 % of our patients report a combination of radicular pains and subsequent paresis within a time window of 48 days. It is only in a comparatively small group of patients that neuroborreliosis is characterized by other symptoms, such as progressive disturbances of gait, organic psychosyndrome, or stroke.

Extraneurological symptoms, apart from cutaneous manifestations (erythema migrans, acrodermatitis chronica atrophicans) and often elevated liver enzyme levels, are rarely observed in Europe. American authors, in contrast, report concomitant arthritis in 24 to 39 % of their patients, and carditis in 4 %.

Syndrome	Germany
Meningoradiculitis cranialis	9 %
Meningoradiculitis spinalis	37 %
Meningoradiculitis cranialis et spinalis	29 %
Meningomyel(oradicul)itis	5 %
Meningoencephal(oradicul)itis	4 %
Meningitis	4 %
Cerebrovascular neuroborreliosis	1 %
Progressive encephalomyelitis	6 %
Mono(poly)neuritis (acute)	3 %
Mono(poly)neuritis (chronic)	2 %

Table 5.3: Neuroborreliosis syndromes in Germany (n = 330)

The individual clinical syndromes of neuroborreliosis occur with variable frequency (☞ Table 5.3) and are described in the sections below.

5.1.2.2.1. Meningoradicul(oneur)itis (stage II, Garin-Bujadoux-Bannwarth syndrome)

Meningoradiculoneuritis, described by *Garin* and *Bujadoux* in 1922 and by *Bannwarth* in 1941 and 1944, is the most common neurological manifestation of neuroborreliosis in Europe, affecting 74 to 86 % of all patients. Various courses have been described.

Meningoradiculitis spinalis

Spinal meningoradiculitis is the classical variant and is observed mainly in older people. The illness usually starts with erythema migrans (38 %) or (pseudo)radicular pains (52 %). Fever and headaches are rarely present at the start, with frequencies of 1.8 and 2.4 %, respectively.

> In the course of the illness all those affected suffer excruciating burning, stabbing, or dragging pains, particularly during the night, often accompanied by dysesthesias. The pains can increase in intensity in attacks or waves and almost disappear in the intervals.

Simple analgesics are usually completely ineffective. The patients have not previously experienced comparable pains. The pains lead to substantial sleep disturbances, so a large proportion of patients walk about their home at night or lie in a cold bath to relieve them. The sequelae of days or weeks of sleep deprivation are clear psychoorganic disturbances, with irritability and disturbances of memory, attention, and drive. The clinical picture is often misinterpreted, and a psychosomatic disturbance or a slipped disk is assumed. In consequence, patients often go through an ordeal lasting weeks, with numerous imaging procedures, occasionally going as far as operations on the slipped disk assumed to be responsible. Misdiagnoses are avoidable, as the course of the illness is generally typical. In two-thirds of the patients the pain starts in the region of an existing tick bite, spreads outward from there, and is ultimately most pronounced in the shoulder or lumbar region, radiating into the limbs. As it progresses, dysesthesias (66 %) and pareses (69 %) occur within certain time limits. An isolated pain syndrome may be present in 28 % of the patients at the time of admission. The neurological findings often include damage to several nerve roots, sometimes with reduced or absent muscular reflexes. The pattern of deficits is asymmetric, both in severity and course. Monoradicular courses which could be confused with a radicular compression syndrome are rare, occurring in 4 % of the cases. Lumbosacral roots are affected most often (67 %). About one patient in five has paresis of the abdominal wall. The clinical severity can range from weakening of the reflexes to very severe sensorimotor tetraparesis. Concomitant illnesses such as diabetes mellitus or cancer seem to make severe courses more likely.

Meningoradiculitis spinalis et cranialis

One in two to three patients with spinal meningoradiculitis develops cranial nerve deficits in the form of **meningoradiculitis spinalis et cranialis**. All cranial nerves can be affected. Only involvement of the olfactory nerve has not yet been reported. The facial nerve is usually damaged, in half of the patients bilaterally. Cranial nerve pareses are particularly common when cervicobrachial spinal nerves are affected at the start.

A subclinical involvement of the spinal cord or the brain can be detected in about 10 % of patients by the presence of pathological findings in the electroencephalogram or in the somatosensory evoked potentials. The pathogen-specific immune response is generally well expressed, with antibodies detectable in both the cerebrospinal fluid and serum in three-quarters of the patients. It is important to remember that a negative serum finding does not exclude the diagnosis, because in 20 % of cases antibodies can only be detected in the cerebrospinal fluid.

Differential diagnosis

The most common clinical **differential diagnoses** in meningoradiculitis, along with the radicular compression syndrome, are as follows:

- neuralgic shoulder myotrophy
- diabetogenic polyradiculopathy
- other pathogen-induced forms of radiculitis
- rheumatic polymyalgia with symptoms which are similarly stronger at night
- periarteritis nodosa
- in isolated cases it is necessary to consider the Guillain-Barrè syndrome or even attacks of angina pectoris.

Differential diagnostics are easier if paresis of the cranial nerves is present. In some patients it is only the cranial nerves that are affected.

Meningoradiculitis cranialis

The presence of **cranial meningoradiculitis** is the leading syndrome in children and adolescents. Males are affected twice as often as females. The leading clinical symptom is unilateral or bilateral facial paresis. Diplegia faciei generally develops consecutively, with a median interval of 3 days. Additional cranial nerves are rarely affected. Erythema migrans is only reported in 20 % of the cases. Because of the common absence of concomitant symptoms, differentiation from idiopathic facial nerve paresis is only possible by examining of the cerebrospinal fluid. In rare cases the cerebrospinal fluid can be normal, and it is then only possible to diagnose the disease on the basis of the presence of erythema migrans or by repeating the lumbar puncture. It is known that inflammatory changes occur only after a certain latency period. The history is generally short, so pathogen-specific antibodies are present in low concentrations. To avoid incorrect diagnoses it is advisable to use the more sensitive immunoblot or to check the cerebrospinal fluid again after 2 weeks. At the time of admission, the serum of 42 % of our patients, and the cerebrospinal fluid of 28 % of them, gave negative antibody findings in the polyvalent ELISA. *Borrelia* infection is responsible for 30 % of facial nerve pareses in children and for 1 to 10 % of those in adults. Depending on the average age of the population examined, the incidence of the cranial meningoradiculitis syndrome is between 5 and 48 % of all cases of neuroborreliosis. The most common **differential diagnosis** is idiopathic facial nerve paresis and, in older patients, diabetic cranial mononeuropathy. Other pathogen-induced diseases (e.g. herpes zoster, mumps, tuberculosis), meningeal neoplasias, sarcoidosis, or internistic systemic diseases (systemic lupus erythematosus) rarely come into question.

■ Case history — meningoradiculitis spinalis et cranialis

A 59-year-old patient came to admission and reported that he had been suffering from extremely severe burning and racking pains of varying intensity, which were distinctly worse at night, for about 4 weeks. The focus was in the region of the lower back, spreading into the legs and left arm. Since the onset of the pain he had hardly been able to sleep, and had attempted to obtain relief with cold water or night-time walks. He had visited a number of doctors, who treated him for lumbago using mud baths, massages, and medication, but even the strongest analgesics had not helped. During the last 5 days he had noticed increasing weakness in the left arm. On the day of admission liquid was running out of the left corner of his mouth while he was drinking. The clinical and neurological examination showed an agitated, pain-ridden patient in distinctly impaired general condition, with peripheral facial nerve paresis on the left and moderate peripheral paresis of the left brachial and extensor carpi muscles and with absent biceps and radial reflexes. The Lasègue sign was positive on both sides at 60°. Hyperpathia was present in thoracic segments Th3-11. The chemical laboratory findings showed slightly increased GPT and γ-GT. The CSF count showed lymphoplasmacytic pleocytosis, with 580 cells/µl. Total protein was 1.8 g/l and there was a marked disturbance of the blood-brain barrier (albumin quotient: 35) and intrathecal IgM and IgG synthesis (IgM$_{loc}$: 38 mg/l; IgG$_{loc}$: 10 mg/l). The oligoclonal bands were positive. Both the immunoblot and ELISA showed *Borrelia*-specific antibody synthesis in the cerebrospinal fluid and serum. The EMG showed marked spontaneous activity in the characteristic muscles of C6 and C7 on the left. Neuroborreliosis was diagnosed and antibiotic treatment with cefotaxime (3 × 2 g/day) was commenced, together with carbamazepine (2 × 400 mg) for the pain. An increase in the paresis in the left arm, not unusual in neuroborreliosis, occurred during the first few days. The analgesic treatment had to be intensified, using Saroten 75 mg at night. After about a week the patient reported that the pain had become noticeably less severe, and that he was now able to sleep better. The cerebrospinal fluid examination after 14 days showed a clear reduction in the acute parameters (the cell count was now 58/µl, the total protein 0.8 g/l). Intrathecal specific and nonspecific immunoglobulin synthesis was still detected at the same level. When discharged, the patient was free from pain without medication, the belt-like region of hyperpathia in the thorax had disappeared, and only slight facial nerve paresis was still present. The paresis in the left arm, which had become distinctly worse in the interim, had improved slightly. Three months later the facial paresis had completely regressed under intensive physiotherapy, and the paresis of the left arm had declined. The biceps and radial reflexes were absent. The cerebrospinal fluid was normal, apart from nonspecific (oligoclonal bands) and specific (*Borrelia* immunoblot) intrathecal IgG synthesis. The serum gave a marked IgM and IgG immune responses to numerous *Borrelia* antigens. Controls after 6, 9, and 12 months showed a continuing recovery of strength of the left arm. After a year the only residual symptom was the loss of the biceps and radial reflexes. *Borrelia* serology showed a clear IgG reaction with only weak IgM bands in the immunoblot.

5.1.2.2.2. Meningomyel(oradicul)itis (stage II)

Acute *Borrelia* myelitis is rare, occurring in only 3 to 5 % of neuroborreliosis patients. In general it develops over a period of days to 3 weeks from an already present meningoradiculitis. The history is therefore comparable with that of this syndrome. The possibility of secondary spread to the spinal cord occurring as a result of a pronounced inflammatory reaction has been discussed. Cases of primary myelitis are very rare.

> The main clinical signs are spastic parapareses, supranuclear bladder disturbances, or a sensory transverse spinal cord syndrome. As in neurosyphilis (tabes dorsalis), one-third of the patients have posterior cord damage with spinal ataxia.

In mild cases it may only be possible to detect paraspasticity or positive pyramidal tract signs. Diagnostic signs in the neurological findings which are normally detectable are functional disturbances in the cranial or spinal roots. Clinical signs of an inflammatory process are normally absent. The nonspecific (pleocytosis) and pathogen-specific laboratory tests normally yield pathological findings and simplify diagnosis in individual cases. The somatosensory evoked potentials and magnetically evoked potentials usually show pathological changes. The magnetic resonance tomogram can sometimes confirm the inflammatory process.

 Differential diagnosis

Differential diagnosis is simple if attention is paid to the typical development of the disease and to the multifocal damage to peripheral and central neurogenic structures. The condition needs to be distinguished from other pathogen-induced diseases (e.g. herpes zoster) and neural manifestations of collagen disease or vasculitis.

5.1.2.2.3. Meningitis (stage II)

Side by side with cranial meningoradiculitis, isolated meningitis is a typical syndrome in children and adolescents. In a prospective study (n = 256) 16 % of children with lymphocytic meningitis had a *Borrelia* infection. The prevalence of 0 to 3.6 % in adults may be an underestimate because of the common initial seronegativity (approximately 25 % of the cases). Among our patients 4 % suffered from this syndrome.

> The clinical symptoms are characterized by mild to moderate headaches. Meningeal symptoms (stiff neck, vomiting) are rare. Mild fever is present in 30 to 42 % of the cases.

The cerebrospinal fluid syndrome is comparable with that in patients with isolated cranial meningoradiculitis. During differential diagnostics it is particularly important to remember that this is the most common treatable pathogen in cases of aseptic meningitis in central Europe.

■ **Case history — meningitis**

A 24-year-old patient complained of increasing dull oppressive headaches with fever of up to 39° C for a week. He vomited once on the day of admission. He reported a tick bite in the region of the navel three weeks earlier. The clinical and neurological examination showed moderate meningism and erythema migrans about 8 cm across around the navel. The following laboratory parameters were pathological: ESR after Westergren: 24/49 mm, γ-GT: 68 U/l. Lumbar puncture showed lymphocytic pleocytosis with 256 cells/μl and total protein slightly increased to 0.7 g/l with evidence of disturbance of the blood-brain barrier. Intrathecal immunoglobulin synthesis was not present. Serum immunoblot showed strong *Borrelia*-specific IgM bands against the 66 and 41 kd antigens and moderately strong IgG bands against the 60 and 41 kd antigens. The ELISA result was 320 units (normal range: < 170 U). No antibodies were detected in the cerebrospinal fluid. The patient was given 14 days of treatment with 3 × 2 g/day cefotaxime, the headaches disappearing during the first 3 days and the erythema migrans during the first 5 days of this period. At the control examination after 14 days the cell count had fallen considerably, to 31 cells/μl. Intrathecal IgM synthesis could now be detected in the quotient diagram and oligoclonal bands. The immunoblot showed intrathecal synthesis of *Borrelia*-specific antibodies to the 41 kd antigen. The antibody specificity index for IgG was positive, at 1.6. The serum showed an expansion of the antibody pattern, with the detection of numerous *Borrelia*-specific IgM and IgG bands. The ELISA result was 580 units. The patient was discharged in an asymptomatic state, and controls after 3 and 12 months did not reveal any clinical abnormalities. Strong *Borrelia*-specific IgG antibody bands and a weak IgM band could still be detected in the serum after 12 months.

5.1.2.2.4. Meningoencephal(oradicul)itis (stage II)

The frequency of acute *Borrelia* encephalitis is still under discussion. Case reports from the USA in particular do not always satisfy the diagnostic guidelines of European authors. The frequency of this course in our own patients was 4 %. Both children and adults can be affected. The temporal course comprises a prodromal syndrome lasting days or weeks, with fever, myalgias, and headaches leading to progressive symptoms of encephalitis. Spinal meningoradiculitis is rarely present at the onset of the disease. For differential-diagnostic reasons, attention should be paid to the presence of peripheral deficits as well. These can be detected in half of the patients.

> The clinical symptoms include both mild psychoorganic disturbances (emotional lability, tiredness, concentration and memory disturbances) and focal symptoms (hemiparesis, cerebellar ataxia).

The case reports occasionally include descriptions of exogenous psychoses with paranoid-hallucinatory symptoms, catatonia, and depression. Attacks of grand mal, choreoathetosis, and dystonia can occur. We have encountered a Parkinson-like syndrome on three occasions, twice with a clear lateral asymmetry of the rigor and akinesia. The distinguishing signs from idiopathic Parkinson's disease are clinical signs of infection, cranial nerve pareses, and a cerebrospinal fluid which always shows inflammatory alterations. *Borrelia* encephalitis varies in severity from mild to moderate, but life-threatening cases with brainstem encephalitis have also been described. A mild to moderate general change or focal findings characterize the EEG, which is always pathological. Pathological changes in evoked potentials can be helpful in monosymptomatic cases (e.g. Parkinson-like syndrome), providing evidence of generalized neurogenic damage (☞ Fig. 5.6a+b).

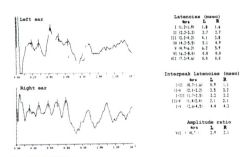

a

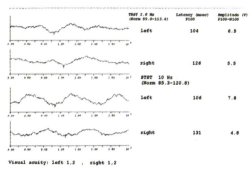

Fig. 5.6a+b: Neurophysiological findings in neuroborreliosis. 53-year-old patient with meningoencephaloradiculitis. **a**: The early auditory evoked potentials (EAEP) show increased interpeak latencies (2-5) as evidence of disturbed brainstem function on the left. **b**: The visual evoked potentials show an increased P-100 latency in demyelinated opticopathy

The cranial MRT and CT are often normal. There have been isolated reports of inflammatory infiltrates, mainly in the medullary center of the cerebellum, stem ganglia, or brainstem. The cerebrospinal fluid is characterized by moderate pleocytosis and pronounced IgM synthesis in comparison with the duration of illness, with a slight disturbance of the blood-brain barrier. Serodiagnostics are made more difficult by the low level of the pathogen-specific immune response in the cerebrospinal fluid.

> The initial detection of antibodies in serum or the detection of a cellular immune response can be indicative. Control puncture generally provides serological confirmation.

In our own experience the common initial seronegativity is easy to reconcile with clinical symptoms which develop very rapidly over a period of days to a maximum of 3 weeks. As in cases of *Borrelia* myelitis, when investigating cases of encephalitis it is important to pay attention to the multifocal neurological findings. Differential diagnosis is similar to that in myelitis, though tuberculosis also needs to be taken into consideration.

■ **Case history — meningoencephalitis**

A 56-year-old woman had increasingly severe dull headaches, exhaustion, and tiredness for 6 weeks, with fever of up to 38.5°C for 3 weeks; she had also had muscle and joint pains. 2 weeks before admission she developed dizziness, nausea, vomiting, and a change in personality. The acute syndrome leading to admission was an attack of grand mal. During the neurological examination the patient was somnolent, in a distinctly impaired general condition, and displayed meningism and an organic psychosyndrome with disturbances of drive and memory. The MRT was normal. The EEG showed moderate general changes and a discontinuous θ-δ focus on the left. The other laboratory parameters, except for an increased ESR of 24/58 mm after Westergren, a CRP of 12.5 mg/dl, and a γ-GT of 59 U/l, were normal. The cerebrospinal fluid showed lymphocytic pleocytosis, with 101 cells/μl, normal total protein, and intrathecal IgG and IgM synthesis. ELISA and immunoblot showed intrathecal synthesis of *Borrelia*-specific antibodies, while the serum gave negative findings according to ELISA and borderline findings according to the immunoblot. The neurological findings normalized during 14 days of antibiotic treatment with 1×2 g ceftriaxone. The EEG improved, with only mild general change now being evident. The nonspecific cerebrospinal fluid parameters were normalizing, with a cell count of 39/μl and only moderate intrathecal IgG synthesis. Immunoblot tests on the serum and cerebrospinal fluid showed an expansion of the specific immune response. The patient remained free of complaints over a 6-month course-observation period. *Borrelia* serology remained positive in both cerebrospinal fluid and serum.

5.1.2.2.5. Cerebrovascular neuroborreliosis (stage II/III)

If acute *Borrelia* encephalitis or meningitis remains untreated it can (in an unknown percentage of cases) develop into progressive encephalomyelitis or cerebrovascular neuroborreliosis. From the gross-pathological point of view these entities correspond to the disease taking a parenchymatous and vasculitic course.

> The history of patients with cerebrovascular neuroborreliosis is characterized by mild symptoms of meningeal irritation, permanent or transient cranial nerve pareses, and slowly progressive cerebral symptoms (personality changes, memory disturbances), before attacks occur after 3-7 months of illness. The attacks can take the form of recurrent transient ischemic attacks in various vascular territories or isolated cerebral infarcts.

The syndrome is extremely rare. Apart from our own 4 cases, absolute evidence exists for only about another 30 in the literature. The cerebrospinal fluid syndrome is similar to that in progressive encephalomyelitis, though with a distinctly shorter duration of illness. Pathogen-specific antibodies can be detected in the cerebrospinal fluid and serum. CT and MRT show small subcortical infarcts in the capsula interna and the stem ganglia or brainstem (☞ Fig. 5.7b).

In one case autopsy showed a thrombosing arteritis of the perforating arteries of A. basilaris and A. cerebri anterior, with direct spread of the inflammatory process from the meninges. Isolated *B. burgdorferi*-like spirochetes have occasionally been found in the leptomeninges and in the subependymal vessel region. Arteritis of the major vessels may be present, as confirmed by 3 cases of occlusion of A. basilaris. Smaller and medium-sized vessels seem to be the main ones affected, as in Heubner's endarteritis in neurosyphilis. This explains the frequent absence of abnormal angiographic findings.

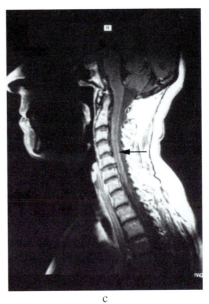

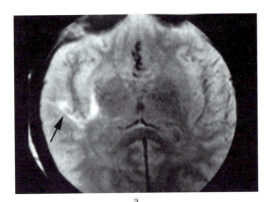

a

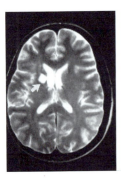 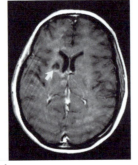

b

c

Fig. 5.7a-c: MRT findings in neuroborreliosis. **a**: 63-year-old man with progressive encephalomyelitis. The cranial MRT (TE 60 ms, TR 2000 ms) provides evidence of increased signal intensity (arrow) in the right medial temporal lobes as an expression of focal encephalitis. **b**: 41-year-old woman with cerebrovascular neuroborreliosis. The cranial MRT (left: TE 80 ms, TR 3000 ms, right: TE 15 ms, TR 650 ms) shows a cerebral infarct in the region of the right caput nuclei caudati, the anterior limb of the capsula interna and the nucleus lentiformis. **c**: 60-year-old woman with progressive encephalomyelitis. The cervical MRT (TE 15 ms, TR 500 ms) after administration of a contrast agent shows a band of increased signal intensity (arrow) as an expression of a disturbance of the blood-brain barrier. (With the kind permission of Prof. Traupe, Neuroradiological Department, Giessen University Hospital)

■ Differential diagnosis

Differential diagnosis is generally easy. Embolic or arteriosclerotic causes can be excluded because of the typical history of meningoencephalitis and the signs of inflammation in the cerebrospinal fluid. Other primary or secondary forms of vasculitis are possible. The *Borrelia* serology, which is always unambiguously positive, is indicative in such cases.

■ Case history — cerebrovascular neuroborreliosis

A 41-year-old woman with clinical symptoms of recurrent ischemic attacks was admitted to hospital in February. She reported attacks of paresis, sometimes on the left and sometimes on the right side of the body for the past 2 months. Up to 6 episodes had sometimes occurred per day, each lasting just a few minutes. Since November she had been suffering the following concomitant symptoms: increased tiredness, poor concentration, dull oppressive headaches, and undirected dizziness. In the preceding few days she had several attacks of vomiting. There were no known vascular risk factors or relevant prior diseases. In October of the previous year she had had erythema migrans. On admission the patient was in impaired general condition. She had lost weight in recent weeks, and appeared weary and exhausted. The clinical and neurological examination showed a mild psychosyndrome with slowness and mnesic disturbances, central facial nerve paresis on the right, increased muscle proprioceptive reflexes on the left, and a large-amplitude static and intentional movement tremor in the upper extremities. At the time of admission the cerebrospinal fluid showed lymphoplasmacytic pleocytosis, with 326 cells/µl, increased protein at 2.45 g/l, and intrathecal IgG synthesis with positive oligoclonal bands after isoelectric focusing. The ESR after Westergren was 15/16 mm. The blood leukocyte count was 8700/µl. Immunoblot and ELISA results (serum 532 U, cerebrospinal fluid 1.169 U, AI: 5.8) confirmed the diagnosis of neuroborreliosis by demonstrating intrathecal IgG synthesis of specific antibodies against *Borrelia* antigens. Cranial MRT revealed an infarct involving the caput nuclei caudati and the anterior limb of the capsula interna (☞ Fig. 5.7b). Cerebral angiography did not reveal anything abnormal. The subjective complaints disappeared after 21 days of treatment with cefotaxime (3 × 2 g daily). The neurological findings normalized. The inflammatory changes in the cerebrospinal fluid were normalizing: cell count 52/µl, total protein 1.42 g/l. After 3 months the patient still had pleocytosis with 36 cells/µl. A further cycle of treatment was carried out with 3 × 2 g/day of cefotaxime for 2 weeks. After a year there was still distinct pleocytosis, with 7 cells/µl, and decreasing intrathecal IgG and IgA synthesis. Specific antibodies in serum could only be detected by the immunoblot technique, no longer with the ELISA. In the cerebrospinal fluid synthesis of specific IgG and IgA antibodies to *Borrelia* antigens was continuing. The MRT was unchanged, with evidence of a cerebral infarct. Clinically, the patient remained asymptomatic from the first discharge until the end of the follow-up tests after 2½ years.

5.1.2.2.6. Progressive encephalomyelitis (stage III)

Progressive encephalomyelitis occurs in stage III of the disease, and was first described by *Ackermann* in 1985. Various authors cite a frequency of between 4.3 and 19 % for this syndrome among patients with neuroborreliosis from collections of case histories. Including our own cases, 92 patients have been reliably documented in the literature. Women and men are affected equally often between the ages of 40 and 60. Cases among children are rare. The duration of illness before diagnosis in these 92 patients was from 6 months to 23 years (median time 14 months). Latency periods between EM and the onset of the disease of between 4 and 12 months have been verified.

> In contrast to acute CNS courses, the history is rarely characterized by a preceding radicular pain syndrome, headaches, or clinical signs of infection. A slowly developing chronic course without pain is characteristic, which may have episodic deteriorations superimposed upon it. Symptom-free intervals have not been described.

As in neurosyphilis, there is a spinal and a cerebral type (tabes dorsalis versus progressive paralysis). The leading symptoms are spastic paraparesis, spinal or cerebellar ataxia, organic psychosyndrome, hemiparesis, or extrapyramidal motor symptoms. The findings can occur in isolation or in combination. Concomitant damage to the spinal roots is observed in 8 to 26 % of the patients. Cranial nerve pareses are about as common as in acute courses, but the predilection is different — the vestibulocochlear nerve is mainly involved in 16 to 80 % of the cases and the optic nerve in 5 to 11 %. The evoked potentials often show pathological changes and can confirm the multifocal character of the disease in monosymptomatic courses (in our own patients: VEP 57 %, FAEP 44 %; ☞ Fig. 5.6). Magnetic resonance tomography shows nonspecific inflammatory changes in the brain or the spinal cord in about half of the patients (☞ Fig. 5.7a+c). The cerebrospinal fluid syndrome is characteristic, with moderate lymphoplasmacytic pleocytosis, marked disturbances of the blood-brain barrier, and often intrathecal synthesis of IgG, IgA, and IgM, allowing a distinction between the acute and chronic courses. Analysis of the cerebrospinal fluid makes it impossible to confuse the condition with multiple sclerosis. It is always possible to detect a pathogen-specific immune response in the cerebrospinal fluid and serum. This facilitates **differential diagnosis** from other inflammatory systemic diseases (e.g. sarcoidosis, systemic lupus erythematodus) that might be considered etiologically because of the chronic multifocal character of tertiary neuroborreliosis.

■ Case history — progressive encephalomyelitis — stage III

In June a 60-year-old woman was admitted to hospital due to an increasing gait disturbance. She reported a gradual decrease in her walking distance over the course of about a year, by then reduced to about 300 meters. She had had a bladder disturbance for about 3 months, often felt unable to hold urine and then had to go quickly to the bathroom. For about 4 weeks she had an ascending sensation of numbness, reaching the level of her navel. The neurological findings included moderate spastic paraparesis of the legs with increased muscle proprioceptive reflexes and positive pyramidal tract signs on both sides, incomplete sensory deficit down from Th10 with disturbances of postural and vibrational perception, spinal ataxia of the legs, and a neurogenic bladder disturbance with a residual urine volume of 200 ml. The ESR was normal, at 5/20 mm after Westergren. The cerebrospinal fluid showed lymphoplasmacytic pleocytosis of 50 cells/µl, an increase in the total protein level to 1.8 g/l, and a pronounced disturbance of the blood-brain barrier with intrathecal IgG synthesis and the detection of oligoclonal bands. Lactate was elevated, at 3.47 mmol/l. The ELISA results for *Borrelia* were 1336 (serum) and 1358 units (cerebrospinal fluid), with an antibody index of 13.8 (for calculation ☞ Section 6.1.3.4.). The immunoblot demonstrated marked local synthesis of *Borrelia*-specific IgG antibodies to numerous *Borrelia* antigens in the cerebrospinal fluid and serum. Only low levels of IgM antibodies were present. There was a slight general change in the EEG and pathological visual evoked potentials, without clinical correlates. The MRT showed a band-shaped barrier disturbance in the region of the cervical spinal cord (☞ Fig. 5.7 c). The patient was diagnosed with serologically confirmed progressive encephalomyelitis and a 3-week course of intravenous antibiotic treatment with 3 × 2 g cefotaxime was started. This led to a continuous, though very slow, improvement in the neurological findings. After 9 months the patient was once more able to walk a few kilometers. Examinations showed only a very mild spastic paraparesis of the legs and a sensible deficit. The spinal ataxia was unchanged. The bladder disturbance had disappeared completely. The cerebrospinal fluid still showed slight pleocytosis, with 8 cells/µl, and a normal total protein level. The positive oligoclonal bands due to a marked intrathecal IgG immune response to numerous *Borrelia* antigens remained unchanged. The EEG had normalized. At the patient's request no further course controls were carried out.

5.1.2.2.7. Lyme encephalopathy

In American literature Lyme encephalopathy is classified among the chronic courses. In this condition disturbances of memory and perception and abnormal tiredness persist after the early stages of Lyme borreliosis (e.g. EM, Lyme arthritis), or the symptoms may develop over the following months or years.

According to the literature the deficits can be measured objectively in neuropsychological tests. The EEG and the cerebrospinal fluid are almost always normal. MRT sometimes shows white matter lesions. The clinical, neurophysiological, and SPECT results improve in some patients under antibiotic treatment. Against the background of European literature it is astonishing to find that the inflammatory signs in the cerebrospinal fluid, including intrathecal synthesis of specific antibodies, are often absent at the time of the diagnosis. This contradicts all previous experience with spirochete infections. It is conceivable that Lyme encephalopathy corresponds to a defect syndrome after subclinical encephalitis, e.g. in acute Lyme arthritis, and is only noticed in everyday life after the acute phase of the disease has subsided. This is supported by the frequent subclinical pathological EEG findings in 29 % of our own patients, and by two autopsies carried out on neuroborreliosis patients. One patient with paraplegic myelitis was found to have disseminated perivascular lymphocytic infiltrates in the brain. No symptoms of brain disease had been present during the patient's lifetime (☞ Fig. 5.8c).

5.1.2.2.8. Acute and chronic neuritis, myositis, and fasciitis (stage II/III)

Isolated neuritis with normal cerebrospinal fluid can occur in the acute (stage I/II) or chronic (stage III) forms. So far a reliable establishment of the diagnosis is only possible in the presence of pathognomonic skin changes (EM, ACA) (☞ Case history in Section 5.1.2.1.3.). The frequency of this syndrome cannot therefore be established. In our own patient population 5 % of neuroborreliosis patients displayed this syndrome. The pattern of neurogenic involvement can vary, on the one hand taking the form of cutaneous neuritis localized in the region of the skin efflorescences and on the other occurring as isolated damage to the peripheral nerves or a plexus far from the site of entry.

In electrophysiological terms the lesions are axonal. Morphologically, it is possible to detect perivascular lymphoid cell infiltrates of the medium-sized and small perineural and endoneural vessels (☞ Fig. 5.8a). Vascular occlusions occur. Marked axonal degeneration can be observed, with only a small amount of demyelination. Symptoms of cutaneous neuritis are displayed by up to 30 % of patients with EM and by 40 to 60 % of those with ACA. In chronic courses it is not just the skin and the nerves that are affected, but also neighboring joints, muscles, and bones. American authors have described a common, usually mild, chronic axonal polyneuropathy without concomitant skin changes in neuroborreliosis patients. Most of these cases lack convincing etiological documentation in terms of the diagnostic criteria used.

On rare occasions, cases of myositis can occur in stage II and III of Lyme borreliosis, either in isolation or in combination with other neurological symptoms. Involvement of clinically healthy muscle is also possible. Histologically, these are cases of interstitial or focal myositis (☞ Fig. 5.8b).

There have been many reports of fasciitis in patients with *B. burgdorferi* infections. The pictures are clinically and histologically similar to eosinophilic fasciitis (Shulmann's syndrome).

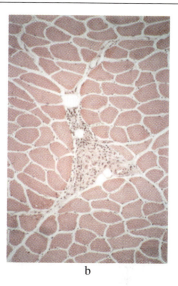

b

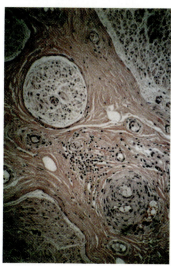

a

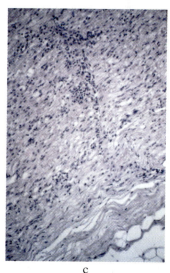

c

Fig. 5.8a-c: Histological findings in neuroborreliosis. **a:** 57-year old patient with meningoradiculitis cranialis et spinalis. The calf biopsy shows interstitial neuritis with perivascularly localized lymphocytic inflammatory cell infiltrates in the epineural, perineural, and endoneural vessels (vasa nervorum). **b:** 76-year old patient with ACA which had been developing for 5 years. The muscle biopsy shows focal lymphoplasmacytic myositis. **c:** 69-year old woman with meningomyeloradiculitis and carditis, who died of a blocked intestine. The autopsy revealed lymphoplasmacytic carditis and numerous lymphoplasmacytic infiltrates, predominantly in the region of the lower spinal cord, in the lumbar spinal ganglia and roots, but also in the brain. (Fig. 5.8a+b: with the kind permission of Prof. Schachenmayr, Neuropathology Institute, Giessen University Hospital)

Differential diagnosis

Borrelia-induced cases of neuritis and myositis are problematic in terms of **differential diagnosis**. Positive serum serology does not constitute unequivocal proof, as this is found in 4 to 7 % of the entire population. A muscle or nerve biopsy with evidence of perivasculitis can be helpful in individual cases. Detection of *Borrelia* in muscle biopsies by culture or by molecular biology methods is possible. Once other possible causes have been ruled out, antibiotic treatment (e.g. with cefotaxime) should be tried even if the pathogen has not been detected directly.

5.1.2.3. Internistic manifestations

Internistic involvements in Lyme borreliosis take the form of the rare acute Lyme carditis and the more common acute to chronic Lyme arthritis. Isolated involvement of the liver, spleen, kidneys, or lungs seems to occur at most in individual cases. According to our own experience, however, up to 40 % of neuroborreliosis patients show a slight reversible increase in GOT, GPT, or γ-GT in the sense of concomitant hepatitis. Proteinuria and macrohematuria are also observed in 6 % of stage II patients. Permanent damage has not been observed. *Borrelia* has been detected histologically in liver or spleen biopsies from individual patients and from the lungs of another patient who had fatal interstitial pneumonia. Animal studies and autopsies of stillborn children have revealed *Borrelia* in the kidneys, liver, brain, adrenals, in the meninges, and in the subarachnoidal space. This suggests the possibility of wide dissemination of the pathogen. In practice, however, only involvement of the heart and the joints is important.

5.1.2.3.1. Lyme arthritis

Lyme arthritis (☞ Fig. 5.9) can occur in stage II or III of the disease. It needs to be distinguished from arthralgias, which are very often reported in stage I (20 to 50 %). The relative frequency of Lyme arthritis in Germany is said to be 8 to 10 % of all cases. Among our own patients with neuroborreliosis the prevalence was 3 %.

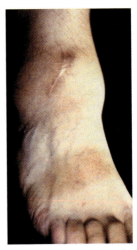

Fig. 5.9: Arthritis of the ankle in Lyme borreliosis (with the kind permission of Dr. Hassler)

According to the CDC, 41 % of all Lyme borreliosis patients reported in the USA between 1990 and 1993 (n = 34 502) had suffered from arthritis. A recently published prospective study in German children gave an incidence of 4/100 000. The arthritis develops with an average latency period of four weeks after erythema migrans, which about 30 to 40 % of the patients were able to recall.

> Clinically, it appears typically in the form of mono- or oligoarthritis; it affects the large joints, and of these preferentially the knee (80 to 94 %).

The ankle, hand, toe, elbow, finger, metatarsal, and heel joints are affected less often. The course of the disease is generally intermittent, being characterized by attacks and remissions. The duration of the individual attacks of arthritis varies from days to months, with an average duration of one week. Between these attacks there are periods of remission lasting from days to weeks. Without treatment, spontaneous remission generally occurs after a median total duration of 6-7 months. About 10 % of the acute Lyme arthritis cases develop into the chronic form (stage III). This is usually preceded by the attacks becoming longer and more intense, with shorter periods of remission. The chronic form loses its intermittent character and mostly affects the knee joint on one or both sides. In children the arthritis, like tertiary neuroborreliosis, can follow a primary chronic progressive form in almost 18 % of the cases. In adults this seems to be less common. Concomitant symptoms of other organ manifestations in children are extremely rare in Europe, while in the USA the figure quoted is over 15 %. Arthritis can occur as a concomitant symptom of acrodermatitis chronica atrophicans (☞ Case history in Section 5.1.2.1.3.). Clinical examination often reveals very pronounced articular effusion with restricted mobility and swelling. Reddening and hyperthermia can occur. The pain symptoms are remarkably few. Baker's cysts are described in up to 10 % of the cases. Chronic cases can lead to joint destruction with ankylosis.

Changes in the laboratory parameters

Of the nonspecific **changes in the laboratory parameters**, a moderate increase in the erythrocyte sedimentation rate in 80 % of children and 50 % of adults is striking. In the acute stage of the arthritis arthrocentesis reveals polymorphonuclear leukocytosis, with 26 000 cells/μl (range 500 to 110 000/μl) and an increased protein concentration (3 to 8 g/dl). Immune complexes are regularly detected.

Synovial biopsy

Synovial biopsy of chronic forms reveals villose hypertrophy, fibrin deposits, neovascularization, and lymphoplasmacytic infiltrates. The changes are nonspecific and may also be observed e.g. in rheumatoid arthritis.

Radiological findings

Radiology shows soft-tissue changes in the acute stage and loss of cartilage, subchondral cysts, and juxta-articular osteoporosis together with cortical bone erosions in the chronic phase. Lyme arthritis does not differ clinically from other acute forms of arthritis.

Differential diagnosis

In **differential diagnosis** it is necessary to look at the possibility of arthropathies caused by crystal formation, such as gout or chondrocalcinosis, reactive forms of arthritis such as Reiter's syndrome, and enteropathic forms of arthritis. Löfgren's syndrome (bilateral hilar lymphoma syndrome), psoriatic arthritis, and reactivated arthrosis also need to be borne in mind. Symmetrical involvement of the small joints is not typical, so in differential diagnostics rheumatoid arthritis would only be a possibility if it followed an atypical course.

5.1.2.3.2. Lyme carditis

Involvement of the heart can occur in the first week of infection and should be classified as stage II. Its frequency is said to be 8 % in the USA and 0.2 to 3.3 % in Europe. Concomitant neurological and dermatological symptoms are often reported. It is unclear whether it was these complaints that had led to the diagnosis, or whether carditis is generally more common in severe courses with oligosymptomatic involvement of organs. The most common clinical complaints are conduction disturbances, especially alternation between 1st and 3rd-degree AV blocks, as well as atrial fibrillation and intraventricular conduction disturbances with extrasystoles. As a rule the cardiac symptoms only last a short time (3 days to 6 weeks) and are very well reversible. Severe courses with dilative cardiomyopathy and, in one case with a fatal pancarditis, are rare. **Histology** shows perivascular lymphoplasmacytic infiltrates in the myocardium, pericardium, and endocardium.

5.1.2.4. Ophthalmoborreliosis

In 1985 *Steere* first reported microscopic detection of spirochetes in the eyes of a woman who developed severe panophthalmitis 4 weeks after erythema migrans. Since that time manifestations of Lyme borreliosis have been observed and described in all parts of the eye. The eye can be affected primarily or it can become a secondary target due to infection of its adnexa (e.g. lagophthalmic keratitis in facial nerve paresis). Primary ophthalmic manifestations are possible in all three stages. In stage I, migration of the erythema over the eye can lead to conjunctivitis. In stage II all parts of the eye can be affected. Case histories describe chorioretinitis (☞ Fig. 5.10), iridocyclitis, ocular myositis, and keratitis as ophthalmological manifestations.

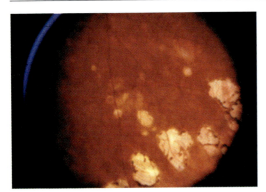

Fig. 5.10: Chorioretinitis in Lyme borreliosis. 24-year-old woman with EM, chorioretinitis, and paralysis of the inner oculomotor nerves. Ophthalmoscopy shows multiple chorioretinal inflammatory foci

In addition to paralysis of the inner and outer ocular muscles, inflammation of the optic nerve is encountered in 1 to 3 % of the patients with neurological symptoms. From time to time a unilateral or bilateral papilledema is observed even though the patient has not reported any complaints. Pathological visual evoked potentials can be detected in up to 25 % of patients with stage III neuroborreliosis. Bilateral keratitis 5 years after the onset of Lyme arthritis has been reported in an 11-year-old girl. Ophthalmoborreliosis can occur in isolation or in combination with other extraocular manifestations of Lyme borreliosis. The exact frequency of this form of the disease is unknown, as the described forms of intraocular inflammation are not pathognomonic. In the absence of erythema migrans or serologically established neuroborreliosis, the only methods left in these cases are the collection of biopsies or detection of *Borrelia*-specific antibodies in the aqueous humor. Since this can rarely be done in practice, the question of association cannot be answered definitely in most cases.

■ **Case history — ophthalmo- and dermatoborreliosis — stage II**

A 24-year old woman reported a typical picture of erythema migrans about 10 days after a tick bite. The EM disappeared under 2 weeks of oral treatment with 200 mg/day of doxycycline. At the end of the antibiosis the patient experienced increasing dull headaches and visual disturbances on the right. As the complaints did not subside, she reported to our special Lyme borreliosis service. The findings indicated paresis of the inner ocular muscles and florid chorioretinitis on the right-hand side (☞ Fig. 5.10). The cerebrospinal fluid and the other laboratory parameters in the serum were normal. The *Borrelia* ELISA result in serum was 280 units (limit: 180 U). The immunoblot revealed specific IgM bands against the 61, 41, and 12 kd antigens and IgG bands against the 75, 41, and 35 kd antigens. Lyme borreliosis was diagnosed and treatment with 20 MU penicillin G was commenced. After 14 days there was a strong *Borrelia*-specific immune response, with an ELISA result of 850 units, specific IgM antibodies to the 66, 60, 41, 30, 15, and 12 kd antigens, and IgG antibodies to the 75, 66, 60, 41, and 35 kd antigens. The paresis of the inner ocular muscles and the chorioretinitis slowly regressed over the course of 3 months.

5.2. Tick-borne encephalitis

5.2.1. Course of the disease

The probability of developing TBE after a tick bite in an area where it is endemic is very difficult to estimate. The most important criteria for risk assessment are the rate of tick infection with the TBE virus and the rate of manifestation of the infection. The rate of tick infection with the TBE virus varies between 0.1 and 5 %, depending on the risk area assessed and on the method of detection (isolation of the virus, PCR). Little is known about the *manifestation rate* of TBE after an infection, but on the basis of earlier studies the manifestation rate is usually said to be 10-30 %.

5.2. Tick-borne encephalitis

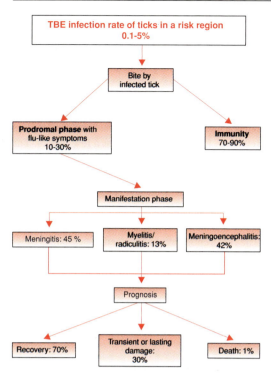

Fig. 5.11: Course of the infection in tick-borne encephalitis

According to more recent studies, however, a substantially higher manifestation rate after infection (approx. 50 %) should be assumed instead (☞ Fig. 5.11)

5.2.1.1. Prodromal phase

The *incubation period*, i.e. the interval between infection (tick bite) and the onset of the first clinical symptoms, is on average between 7 and 14 days. Reports of shorter (3 days) or substantially longer (28 days) incubation periods should be viewed skeptically, as the latter eventuality can be only regarded as credible if the patient visited the risk area only once in the preceding 4 weeks and was on that occasion bitten by a tick. One possible explanation for occasional incubation times which appear to be longer than 2 weeks is the biphasic course of TBE, which is observed in more than 70 % of patients. Both the prodromal phase and the asymptomatic interval between the prodromal and manifestation phases can last up to a week. If the prodromal phase passes unnoticed, the onset of the disease will be defined by the manifestation phase, resulting in a correspondingly longer incubation period.

Influenza-like complaints usually develop during the *prodromal phase* (1 to 2 weeks after the tick bite): patients complain of general malaise, with increasing tiredness, headaches, neck, muscle, and limb pains, and occasional eye pain taking the form of a sensation of retrobulbar pressure. Gastrointestinal complaints such as nausea, vomiting, stomach ache, and diarrhea are occasionally in the foreground instead. The body temperature in this phase is generally increased, to values up to 38°C. Despite the absence of signs of meningeal irritation, the headaches during the prodromal phase can be misinterpreted as meningitis (☞ Table 5.4). Analysis of the cerebrospinal fluid at this time does not, however, show any inflammatory changes and the serology is still negative. The only abnormal laboratory parameters observed are leukopenia, thrombopenia and sometimes elevation of liver

Prodromal stage	Manifestation stage
• General malaise	• *Meningitis* Headaches, fever, stiff neck, nausea, vomiting
• Headaches, limb pains, fever	• *Encephalitis* Quantitative and qualitative disturbances of consciousness, cranial nerve pareses [III, IV, VI, VII, VIII, IX, X, XI, XII], disturbances of balance and dizziness, hemipareses, epileptic fits, vegetative regulation disturbances, central respiratory and circulatory regulation disturbances, disturbances of concentration and memory, tremor
• Gastrointestinal complaints such as nausea, diarrhea	• *Myelitis/radiculitis* Proximally emphasized monopareses and parapareses, tetrapareses, bladder voiding disturbances, radicularly distributed sensitivity disturbances

Table 5.4: Disease stages in TBE

enzymes. This first phase of illness lasts only a few days (1-8) and is usually followed by an asymptomatic interval lasting on average a week (4-14 days).

5.2.1.2. Manifestation phase

The second phase of the disease usually begins abruptly, with severe headaches and a clear increase in temperature (☞ Table 5.4). Depending on the size of the study and the diagnostic criteria, the infection of the nervous system manifests itself in the following ways:

- 43-55 % as isolated meningitis
- 40-50 % as meningoencephalitis
- 10-15 % as meningoencephalomyelitis or meningoencephaloradiculitis.

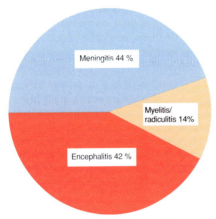

Fig. 5.12: Frequency distribution of the individual forms of manifestation of TBE in 656 patients who fell ill in Baden-Württemberg between 1994 and 1998

The casuistics relating to the period between 1994 and 1997 in Baden-Württemberg showed isolated meningitis and meningoencephalits to be roughly equally common (☞ Fig. 5.12).

5.2.2. Organ manifestations and syndromes

5.2.2.1. Meningitis

■ Clinical symptoms

The courses involving meningitis are often dominated by headaches concentrated in the occipital or fronto-occipital region. The meningism itself is of variable severity and can occasionally be absent. Compared with other viral forms of meningitis, the fever is usually very high, as a rule with temperatures up to 40°C. In the acute stage the patients suffer from increased photosensitivity, dizziness, nausea, and vomiting. In isolated cases there may be transient isolated pareses of the facial and abducent nerves. The acute meningitis persists for about 5-8 days, followed by disappearance of the nausea and fever. The headaches can persist for a few days longer, sometimes for a few weeks. The average period of hospitalization is 10 days (1-30). Overall, the meningitis has a good prognosis and usually clears up without sequelae.

■ Differential diagnosis

The differential diagnosis needs to consider other forms of aseptic meningitis (particularly those caused by infection with enteroviruses, type 2 herpes simplex virus, the varicella-zoster virus, and the mumps virus) and occasionally also septic (bacterial) forms of meningitis (*Listeria monocytogenes, Streptococcus pneumoniae, Haemophilus influenzae, Neisseria meningitidis*).

■ Case history — meningitis

A 17-year-old girl from Dreisam Valley near Freiburg was admitted to hospital due to severe headaches, dizziness, vomiting, and a temperature of 40°C. One week before admission she had already had severe headaches and diarrhea lasting 3 days. She did not remember a tick bite.

At the initial examination the patient was in distinctly impaired general condition. There was tenderness in the epigastrium. Apart from slight pain when bending the neck, the neurological examination did not reveal anything abnormal. The peripheral blood showed distinct leukocytosis, with 19 000 cells/µl, the erythrocyte sedimentation rate according to Westergren was only slightly increased, at 13 mm in the first hour. Analysis of the cerebrospinal fluid showed 45 cells/µl, of which 70 % were granulocytes, 10 % monocytes, and 20 % lymphocytes, and an increased total protein level of 620 mg/l (albumin quotient: 10×10^{-3}).

Investigation of the abdominal complaints by ultrasonography and diagnostic imaging did not reveal anything abnormal. A rapid improvement in the general condition occurred under symptomatic treatment. The fever, headaches, and dizziness reversed within 5 days. After a total of 10 days of treatment the patient was discharged in an asymptomatic state.

Serology confirmed the suspected TBE. Both IgM and IgG antibodies to TBE were positive in the serum. Intrathecal synthesis of specific antibodies was not detected at the time of admission.

5.2.2.2. Encephalitis

Clinical symptoms

Meningoencephalitis differs from isolated meningitis by the additional occurrence of disturbances of consciousness, focal neurological signs and/or changes in the EEG. The course of the disease is more serious, the fever and neurological symptoms generally lasting longer than in meningitis. Many patients are drowsy or somnolent for a few days, in cases which progress rapidly soporific or comatose disturbances of consciousness may be observed. Qualitative disturbances of consciousness are less common, and usually express themselves in the form of delirious states with locational, temporal, and situative disorientation, states of excitation and confusion, and (rarely) optical hallucinations as well.

As shown by autopsy studies from earlier years, replication of TBE viruses takes place in the brain, preferentially in the medulla oblongata, pons, mesencephalon, diencephalon, cortex, Purkinje cells in the cerebellum, and the cervical spinal cord. In the brainstem it is mainly the nuclei of the motor cranial nerves which are affected, and cells of the anterior horn in the spinal cord. The clinical deficits can be well explained on the basis of this pattern. Dizziness is one of the complaints which is often reported, and is usually associated clinically with pronounced ataxia. This is occasionally so severe that the patient is unable to walk. Other symptoms which point toward a brainstem infection are pareses of the ocular muscles, the facial nerve, the vestibulocochlear nerve, and the caudal cranial nerves, with marked disturbances of speech and the ability to swallow. Disturbances of the vegetative regulation of respiration and circulation are associated with the risk of sudden death, and usually observed in rapidly progressive forms. The various forms of nystagmus (gaze, downbeat, or directional nystagmus) and tremor (intentional, static, or resting tremor) can be explained by different forms of anatomical damage. Along with choreiform movement disturbances, occasional patients show rigor-like increase in muscular tone, which in combination with hypokinesia or bradydiadochokinesia and resting tremor, suggests an involvement of the extrapyramidal system. Patients with TBE sometimes present with aphasic disturbances, a hemiparesis, and focal or generalized attacks. Concentration, memory, and drive are substantially impaired during the acute phase of the disease. Encephalitis patients are generally treated in hospital for an average of 15 days (6-70 days).

Differential diagnosis

Depending on the clinical symptoms, differential diagnosis may need to exclude listeriosis, herpes simplex virus, varicella zoster virus, or enteroviral encephalitis.

■ Case history — meningoencephalitis

The 54-year-old patient had last had a complete active inoculation against TBE 5 years earlier. During a holiday in Kinzigtal he received multiple tick bites. One week before hospital admission he had had headaches and muscle pains, slight fever, episodes of vomiting, and severe diarrhea for a few days. After 3 days of improvement he once more experienced fever, severe headaches, and double vision.

At the initial examination his body temperature was 39.2°C and his general condition was distinctly impaired. The clinical findings were mild meningism, a horizontal gaze nystagmus and abducent nerve paresis. Otherwise his neurological status was normal. Within 2 days he developed pronounced unsteadiness when standing or walking and was no longer able to get out of bed. His consciousness was distinctly clouded, and he spent most of the day sleeping. The abducent nerve paresis and gaze paresis regressed after 5 days. From the ninth day the patient was once more alert and his temperature had normalized. Although the ataxia gradually regressed, it was still present in a mild form at the time of discharge on day 14: he still could not walk in a straight line or stand on one leg.

At the follow-up examination three months after discharge the patient was asymptomatic.

At the time of admission the inflammation parameters in the peripheral blood were distinctly elevated: leukocytes 15 000/µl; ESR after Westergren 34 mm; CRP 5 mg/dl. TBE serology was unambiguously positive. Analysis of the cerebrospinal fluid on the day of admission showed 143 cells/µl, of which 40 % were granulocytes, 30 % monocytes, and 30 % lymphocytes, and a slight disturbance of the blood-brain barrier (total protein 830 mg/l, albumin quotient 14×10^{-3}). Intrathecal synthesis of immunoglobulins or TBE antibodies was not detected. In the subsequent examination after one week the cell count had increased to 220/µl (90 % lymphocytes, 10 % monocytes) and the albumin quotient to 20×10^{-3}. In addition, by that time there was intrathecal synthesis of total IgM (40 %) and IgG (10 %) and of TBE-specific IgM and IgG antibodies.

■ Case history — meningoencephalitis

The 72-year-old patient had lived in an TBE risk area since childhood and reported countless tick bites, most recently 3 weeks ago. For 2 days he had severe headaches and a temperature of up to 39°C. He was admitted to hospital because of acute facial nerve paresis and increasing weakness in the right arm and leg.

At the initial examination the patient was somnolent and only capable of limited cooperation, his general condition was distinctly impaired. Apart from the paresis of the facial nerve, the cranial nerve status was normal. There was a central hemiparesis on the right, affecting mainly the arm.

Within a day his clinical condition had deteriorated greatly. The next morning he had two generalized convulsive seizures and the hemiparesis had developed into hemiplegia. On the same day the patient suffered respiratory insufficiency and lost consciousness. He was intubated and transferred to an intensive-care ward. Consciousness returned after 2 weeks in a coma. He then displayed severe pareses of the caudal cranial nerves, tetraparesis of the extremities, and a lack of respiratory drive. After 10 months of treatment in the intensive-care ward the patient died from secondary complications. During this period there was no regression of the pareses or of the respiratory failure. Repeated MRT examinations did not reveal any specific changes.

At the initial examination the leukocyte count was distinctly increased at 18 000/µl, as was the ESR after Westergren, at 41 mm. TBE serology was negative. The cerebrospinal fluid contained 356 cells/µl, of which 80 % were granulocytes and 20 % monocytes. Total protein was moderately increased, at 820 mg/l. Control examinations after 1 and 3 weeks showed distinctly increased antibody titers (IgM and IgG) against the TBE virus. The patient developed a high level of IgM and IgG synthesis in the cerebrospinal fluid, and examination of the CSF 3 weeks after the onset of illness also showed intrathecal synthesis of TBE-specific antibodies (IgM and IgG).

5.2.2.3. Encephalomyelitis and radiculitis

Clinical symptoms

Myelitic courses in TBE almost always occur in association with meningoencephalitis. The neurological symptoms in this course form usually develop very quickly, within hours or days, and generally lead to serious pareses. Mono-, para-, and tetrapareses have been observed, and compared with poliomyelitis these tend to have a proximal distribution, and more often affect the upper extremities than the lower. Since TBE viruses have a particular predilection for cells of the cervical spinal cord, there is a corresponding incidence of tetrapareses and marked paresis of the head levator muscles. In the acute stage the reflexes are generally weakened or absent, in the later course they may continue to be absent (isolated anterior horn infection) or even become hypersensitive (additional involvement of descending pathways). Correspondingly, muscle tone is initially low and later occasionally increased. Loss of sensitivity is the exception in myelitic forms. On the other hand, central bladder disturbances are more common.

In the early stages of the disease **radiculitis** cannot be distinguished from myelitis either on the basis of the paresis distribution pattern or the electrophysiological findings. The segmental distribution of the sensitivity disturbances in radiculitis can be taken as the only possible differential-diagnostic criterion. Pain can occur in both course forms. Unlike myelitis, radiculitis can sometimes occur before the encephalitic symptoms, and in isolated cases it can start at the end of the manifestation phase (after the fever has subsided). The severe pareses in the acute phase are generally followed by pronounced atrophy, particularly in the shoulder muscles (☞ Fig. 5.13).

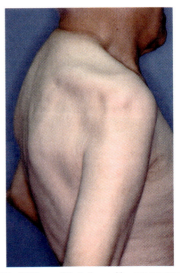

Fig. 5.13: TBE myelitis followed by pronounced muscular atrophy in the shoulder and arm region

The average stay in hospital is longest in the case of myelitis, being 2 months on average (2 weeks to 1 year). All the patients we investigated required inpatient treatment for several weeks or months.

Differential diagnosis

In cases of highly febrile encephalomyelitis the **differential diagnosis** first needs to exclude poliomyelitis, but the associated pareses are more frequent in the lower extremities, where they are usually concentrated in the distal regions. Infections with enteroviruses or varicella-zoster virus also lead to myelitis with similarly severe courses.

5.2.2.4. Manifestations outside the nervous system

In the great majority of cases TBE manifests itself in the central nervous system, but there have been isolated reports of transient hepatitis, pancreatitis, and myocarditits. Within the framework of our own investigations 17 out of 180 patients tested had elevated liver enzymes (GOT, GPT, γ-GT).

References

Ackermann R., Kruger K., Roggendorf M., Rehse-Kupper B., Mortter M., Schneider M. (1986). Vukadinovic I: Spread of early-summer meningoencephalitis in the Federal Republic of Germany. Dtsch. Med. Wochenschr. 111: 927-933

Ackermann R., Rehse-Kupper B., Gollmer E., Schmidt R. (1988). Chronic neurologic manifestations of erythema migrans borreliosis. Ann. N. Y. Acad. Sci. 539: 16-23

Arzneimittelkommission. (1993). Impfung gegen Frühsommer-Meningoenzephalitis: Indikationen - Risiken. Dt. Ärzteblatt. 90: 755

Asbrink. E., Olsson. I. (1985). Clinical manifestations of erythema chronicum migrans Afzelius in 161 patients. A comparison with Lyme disease. Acta. Derm. Venerol. Stockh. 65: 509-514

Bannwarth. H. (1941). Chronische lymphozytäre Meningitis, entzündliche Polyneuritis und Rheumatismus Arch. Psych. Nerv. 113: 284-376

Benke. T., Gasse T., Hittmair-Delazer M., Schmutzhard E. (1995). Lyme encephalopathy: long-term neuropsychological deficits years after acute neuroborreliosis. Acta. Neurol. Scand. 91: 353-357

Bergloff J., Gasser R., Feigl B. (1994). Ophthalmic manifestations in Lyme borreliosis. A review. J. Neuroophthalmol. 14 (1): 15-20

Blumenthal W., Ackermann R., Schottky A. (1970). Zentraleuropäische Enzephalitis unter dem Bild einer lumbalen Poliomyelitis. Med. Klinik. 65: 153-156

Bodemann H., Hoppe-Seyler P., Blum H., Herkel L. (1980). Schwere und ungünstige Verlaufsformen der Zeckenenzephalitis (FSME) 1979 in Freiburg. Dtsch. Med. Wochenschr. 105: 921-924

Brade V., Burmester G.R. (1990). Klinik und Diagnostik der Lyme Borreliose. Editiones Roche

Christen H.J., Bartlau N., Hanefeld F., Eiffert H., Thomssen R. (1990). Peripheral facial palsy in childhood-Lyme borreliosis to be suspected unless proven otherwise. Acta. Paediatr. Scand. 79 (12): 1219-1224

Christen H.J., Hanefeld F., Eiffert H., Thomssen R. (1993). Epidemiology and clinical manifestations of Lyme borreliosis in childhood. A prospective multi-centre study with special regard to neuroborreliosis. Acta. Paediatr. Suppl. 386: 1-75

Duniewicz M. (1976). Klinisches Bild der Zentraleuropäischen Zeckenenzephalitis. Münch. Med. Wschr. 118: 1609-1612

Duray P.H., Steere A.C. (1988). Clinical pathologic correlations of Lyme disease by stage. Ann. N. Y. Acad. Sci. 539: 65-79

Gold R., Wiethoelter H., Rihs I., Löwer J., Kappos L. (1992). Frühsommer-Meningoenzephalitis-Impfung. Indikation und kritische Beurteilung neurologischer Impfkomplikationen. Dtsch. Med. Wochenschr. 117: 112-116

Grinschgl G. (1955). Virus meningoencephalitis in Austria. Clinical features, pathology, and diagnosis. Bull. Wld. Hlth.Org. 12: 535-564

Gunther G., Haglund M., Lindquist L., Forsgren M., Skoldenberg B. (1997). Tick-bone encephalitis in Sweden in relation to aseptic meningo-encephalitis of other etiology: a prospective study of clinical course and outcome. J. Neurol. 244: 230-238

Halperin J., Luft B.J., Volkman D.J., Dattwyler R.J. (1990). Lyme neuroborreliosis. Peripheral nervous system manifestations. Brain. 113 (4): 1207-1221

Halperin J.J., Volkman D.J., Wu P. (1991). Central nervous system abnormalities in Lyme neuroborreliosis. Neurology. 41 (10): 1571-1582

Hansen K., Lebech A.M. (1992). The clinical and epidemiological profile of Lyme neuroborreliosis in Denmark 1985- 1990. A prospective study of 187 patients with *Borrelia burgdorferi* specific intrathecal antibody production. Brain 115 (2): 399-423

Heinz F.X., Ashmera J., Januska J. (1981). Present activity in natural foci of tick-borne encephalitis in the CSSR; in Kunz C (ed): Tick-borne Encephalitis. Vienna, Facultas-Verlag: 279-281.

Herzer P., Wilske B., Preac-Mursic V., Schierz G., Schattenkirchner M., Zollner N. (1986). Lyme arthritis: clinical features, serological, and radiographic findings of cases in Germany. Klin. Wschr.64 (5): 206-215

Hopf H.C. (1975). Peripheral neuropathy in acrodermatitis chronica atrophicans (Herxheimer). J. Neurol. Neurosurg. Psychiatry 38: 452-458

Horst H. (1991). Einheimische Zeckenborreliose (Lyme Borreliose) bei Mensch und Tier Perimed-Fachbuchgesellschaft

Huppertz H.I., Karch H., Suschke H.J., Döring E., Ganser G., Thon A., Bentas W. (1995). Lyme Arthritis in European Children and Adolescents. Arthritis & Rheumatism 3: 361-368

Kaiser R. (1994). Variable CSF findings in early and late Lyme neuroborreliosis: a follow-up study in 47 patients. J. Neurol. 242 (1): 26-36

Kaiser R., Braun H., Dörstelmann D., Hansmann P., von Laer D., Lücking C. H., Wagner K. (1996). Die Frühsommer-Meningoenzephalitis - Beobachtungen zur Klinik und Häufigkeit im Schwarzwald 1994. Akt. Neurologie 23: 21-25

Kaiser R., Kern A., Fressle R., Steinbrecher A., Malzacher V., Kügler D., Kampa D., Batsford S., Omran H. (1996). Zeckenvermittelte Erkrankungen in Baden-Württemberg: Epidemiologische Studie zur Häufigkeit stationär behandlungsbedürftiger FSME- und Borreliose-Erkrankungen im Jahr 1995. Münch. Med. Wschr. 138: 647-652

Kock T., Stunzner D., Freidl W., Pierer K. (1992). Clinical aspects of early summer meningoencephalitis in Styria. Nervenarzt 63: 205-208

Kohlhepp W., Kuhn W., Kruger H. (1989). Extrapyramidal features in central Lyme borreliosis. Eur. Neurol. 29 (3): 150-155

Kohlhepp W., Mertens H.G., Oschmann P., Rohrbach E. (1987). Acute and chronic diseases in transmitted borreliosis by tick bite. Nervenarzt 58 (9): 557-563

Krausler J. (1981). 23 years of TBE in the district of Neunkirchen (Austria). In: Kunz C. (ed): Vienna, Facultas-Verlag

Kruger H-. Reuss K-. Pulz M., Rohrbach E., Pflughaupt K.W., Martin R., Mertens H.G. (1989). Meningoradiculitis and encephalomyelitis due to *Borrelia burgdorferi*: a follow-up study of 72 patients over 27 years. J. Neurol. 236 (6): 322-328

Kruger H., Kohlhepp W., Konig S. (1990). Follow-up of antibiotically treated and untreated neuroborreliosis. Acta Neurol. Scand. 82 (1): 59-67

Kuntzer T., Bogousslavsky J., Miklossy J., Steck A., Janzer R., Regli F. (1991). Borrelia rhombencephalomyelopathy. Arch. Neurol. 48 (8): 832-836

Kunz C. (1992). Tick-borne encephalitis in Europe. Acta Leiden. 60: 1-14

Lesser R.L., Kornmehl E.W., Pachner A.R., Kattah J., Hedges T.R., Newman N.M., Ecker P.A., Glassman M.I. (1990). Neuro-ophthalmologic manifestations of Lyme disease. Ophthalmology 97 (6): 699-706

Meurers B., Kohlhepp W., Gold R., Rohrbach E., Mertens H.G. (1990). Histopathological findings in the central and peripheral nervous systems in neuroborreliosis. A report of three cases. J. Neurol. 237 (2): 113-116

Miklossy J., Kuntzer T., Bogousslavsky J., Regli F., Janzer R.C. (1990). Meningovascular form of neuroborreliosis: similarities between neuropathological findings in a case of Lyme disease and those occurring in tertiary neurosyphilis. Acta Neuropathol. Berlin 80 (5): 568-572

Moritsch H., Krausler J. (1957). Die endemische Frühsommer-Meningo-Enzephalo-Myelitis im Wiener Becken ("Schneidersche Krankheit"). Wien. Klin. Wschr. 69: 921

Mosuni M. S., Kaiser R., Motamedi S., Spöttl F. (1974). Frühsommer-Meningoenzephalitis im Bezirk Schärding in den Jahren 1972 und 1973. Wien. Klin. Wschr. 86: 593-596

Oschmann P., Dorndorf W., Wellensiek H.J., Hornig C., Pflughaupt K.W. (1998). Stages and syndromes of Neuroborreliosis. J. Neurol. 245: 262-272

Oschmann P., Hornig C.R., Dorndorf W. (1993). Zerebrovaskuläre Neuroborreliose. Akt. Neurol. 20: 203-206

Pfister H.W., Einhaupl K.M., Preac-Mursic V., Wilske B., Schiere G. (1984). The spirochetal etiology of lymphocytic meningoradiculitis of Bannwarth (Bannwarth Syndrome). J. Neurol. 231: 141-144

Rehse-Kupper B., Danielova V., Klenk W., Abar B., Ackermann R. (1978). The Isolation of Central European Encephalitis (TBE) virus from Ixodes ricinus ticks in southern Germany. Zbl. F. Bakt. Mikrob. u. Hyg. (A). 242: 148-155

Reik L.Jr. (1991). Lyme Disease and the Nervous System. Thieme Verlag

Reisner H. (1981). Clinic and Treatment of Tick-Borne Encephalitis (TBE). In: Kunz C. (ed): Tick-Borne Encephalitis. International Symposium. Vienna, Baden, Facultas: 1-5

Roggendorf M., Goldhofer E., Heinz F.X., Epp C., Deinhardt F. (1981). Frühsommer-Meningoenzephalitis in Süddeutschland - Epidemiologische Untersuchungen. Münch. Med. Wschr. 123: 1407-1411

Roggendorf M., Neumann-Haefelin D., Ackermann R. (1989). Prophylaxe der Frühsommer-Meningoenzephalitis. Dt. Ärzteblatt. 86: A1992-1998

Schaltenbrand G. (1962). Radikulomyelitis nach Zeckenbiß. Münch. Med. Wschr. 104: 829-834

Smith L.G., Pearlman M., Smith L.G., Faro S. (1991). Lyme-Disease: A Review with Emphasis on the Pregnant Woman. Obstetrical and Gynecological Survey 46: 125-130

Steere A.C., Grodzicki R.L., Kornblatt A.N., Craft J.E., Barbour A.G., Burgdorfer W., Schmid G.P., Johnson E., Malawista S.E. (1983). The spirochetal etiology of Lyme disease. N. Engl. J. Med. 308 (13): 733-740

Steere A.C., Malawista S.E., Hardin J.A., Ruddy S., Askenase W., Andiman W.A. (1977). Erythema chronicum migrans and Lyme arthritis. The enlarging clinical spectrum. Ann. Intern. Med. 86 (6): 685-698

Steere A.C., Schoen R.T., Taylor E. (1987). The clinical evolution of Lyme arthritis. Ann. Intern. Med. 107 (5): 725-731

van der Linde M.R. (1991). Lyme carditis: clinical characteristics of 105 cases. Scand. J. Infect. Dis. Suppl. 77: 81-84

Ziebart-Schroth A. (1972). Frühsommer-Meningoenzephalitis (FSME). Klinik und besondere Verlaufsformen. Wien.Klin. Wschr. 84: 778-781

Diagnostics

6. Diagnostics

6.1. Lyme borreliosis

6.1.1. Cardinal symptoms and instrumental examinations

Contrary to numerous literature reports from the USA and elsewhere, most patients with Lyme borreliosis show a characteristic disease picture. The tentative clinical diagnosis is therefore simple if the doctor is familiar with the typical syndromes and their courses (☞ Chapter 5. and Tables 6.1-6.3).

Neuroborreliosis (stage II/III)
• Frequency 10-12 % (Europe)
• Principal cardinal symptom: (pseudo-)radicular pain, worse at night
• Sequential onset of pains, sensitivity disturbances and pareses
• Polytopically distributed focal neurological deficits with emphasis on the peripheral nervous system
• Spontaneous remission with regression of defects (about 30 %), after months in most cases
• Primary or secondary chronic progressive courses (stage III) occur in roughly 1 patient in 10. A painless course involving mainly the central nervous system is typical
• The occurrence of encephalopathic pictures with no detectable inflammatory changes is questionable

Table 6.1: Characteristics of neuroborreliosis (stage II/III)

Lyme arthritis (stage II/III)
• Frequency 8-10 % (Germany)
• Acute onset (weeks to months after the infection)
• Episodic-remitting course lasting weeks (more common) to years (rare) is seen in most cases. Primary chronic progressive courses are rare
• Duration of episodes: from a few days to months, a week on average, with remissions lasting days to weeks
• Mono- or oligoarthritis (knee joint affected in 80-94 % of cases)
• Transition from acute arthritis (stage II) to a chronic progressive form (stage III) is possible in about 10 % of cases
• Apart from erythema migrans, concomitant extrarheumatological symptoms are rare
• Joint effusions with swelling, erythema and warmth are clinically conspicuous. Pain is strikingly mild

Table 6.2: Characteristics of Lyme arthritis (stage II/III)

Lyme carditis (stage II)
• Frequency 0.2-3 % (Europe)
• Acute onset in the first few weeks after infection
• Frequently accompanied by oligosymptomatic organ involvement
• Duration is usually short (3 days to 6 weeks)
• Conduction disturbances with 1st and 3rd degree AV block, atrial flutter, and intraventricular conduction disturbances are clinically conspicuous

Table 6.3: Characteristics of Lyme carditis (stage II)

In rare cases, however, borreliosis may also lead to uncharacteristic symptoms. Forms with a tertiary course are particularly easy to misinterpret on account of their slow and less dramatic progression. In patients with uncharacteristic symptoms a clinical examination focussing on the cardinal symptoms is advisable, together with instrumental diagnostics. If no organ damage is detectable objectively, Lyme borreliosis is unlikely.

> Subjective symptoms alone are an insufficient basis for a diagnosis, even if the blood is seropositive for *Borrelia*. Detectable organ damage, e.g. to the skin, joints, the heart, eyes, or the nervous system must always be present.

It is important to note that about 95 % of all *Borrelia* infections are asymptomatic, the proportion of the population becoming ill depending on age, exposure, and geographic area. At the special Lyme borreliosis clinic at Giessen University Neurological Clinic, for example, manifest illness can be confirmed in only about 5 % of the patients with positive *Borrelia* serology in the winter as opposed to about 20 % in the summer. The remaining patients prove to be cases of 'serum scars' or false positive serological findings. Thus, positive *Borrelia* serology is always just a suggestion, never confirmation, of a connection between antibody detection and disease. Only confirmation of intrathecal synthesis of antibodies in the CSF has a high diagnostic specificity for neuroborreliosis, though extremely rarely even this finding is encountered in clinically healthy individuals (☞ Section 6.1.3.5.). In the absence of acute inflammatory changes (e.g. elevated cell counts) the detection of specific intrathecal antibody synthesis should be interpreted as a "CSF scar" of a nervous system infection which occurred some time ago and was subclinical or was accompanied by only minor symptoms (e.g. wrongly attributed to a slipped disc). It is interesting to note that detection of *Borrelia* in the CSF or urine has been reported in otherwise healthy individuals in isolated cases.

In view of these diagnostic difficulties, diagnostic criteria have been drawn up by the Center of Disease Control in the USA and by a European Consensus Conference for Lyme borreliosis. The American guidelines are intended mainly for epidemiological purposes and are therefore unsuitable for everyday clinical practice. For further information the literature should be consulted. In our experience the diagnostic criteria for neuroborreliosis presented in Table 6.4 have proved very reliable.

Diagnostic criteria for neuroborreliosis	
I	• Neurological syndromes of unknown etiology • CSF cell count above 4/µl • Specific intrathecal antibody synthesis against *Borrelia burgdorferi*
II	• Spinal and/or cranial radiculitis (Bannwarth syndrome) • CSF cell count above 50/µl, total protein > 0.5 g/l, and intrathecal immunoglobulin synthesis • Positive *Borrelia burgdorferi* serology in serum
III	• ECM (diameter > 5 cm) or ACA • Onset of peripheral neurological syndrome and or dermatoborreliosis confirmed by a doctor within an interval of 2 months • Positive *Borrelia burgdorferi* serology in serum

Table 6.4: Diagnostic criteria for neuroborreliosis. The diagnosis can be established if any of the criteria I-III are met

In everyday practice the best practical approach in the clinical evaluation of patients with suspected Lyme borreliosis is to question them about typical symptom constellations (☞ Section 5.1.), focussing on the most frequent cardinal symptom, i.e. on erythema migrans. This occurs in about ¾ of the patients, either in isolation or as an initial phase of the illness. By the time stages II and III have been reached the erythema is generally no longer present, and explicit questioning about it is therefore necessary. In differential diagnostics it is important to distinguish insect sting reactions; here the delay between the tick bite and the onset of erythema and the maximum size of the erythema are helpful (☞ Chapter 5.). Detection of the tick bite is possible in only about 40 % of patients and so is of secondary importance. In contrast to spring-summer encephalitis, there are no endemic areas for Lyme borreliosis, so that geographic information about recent leisure activities or professional duties is unhelpful. The disease can be acquired anywhere, even in prison, as is evident from the medical history of a recently investigated convict with neuroborreliosis meningoradiculitis. The greatest seasonal risk is associated with tick activity in the summer months — consequently, the diagnosis should be borne in mind in the warmer months in particular. Documentation of the case history and physical examination should be followed by specific **additional investigations** focussing on constellations of findings typical of the disease. On suspicion of neuroborreliosis neurophysiological methods (e.g. electromyography or electroneurography) can be used to detect a multifocal involvement of the peripheral and central nervous system. Pathological findings with no clinical correlates (e.g. EEG 30 %) are not uncommon (☞ Table 6.5).

Frequency of pathological findings in neuroborreliosis stages II and III	
Electroencephalogram	28 %
Visual evoked potentials	26 %
Auditory evoked potentials	26 %
Somatosensory evoked potentials	63 %
Electromyography	65 %
Electroneurography	56 %
Computed tomography	8 %
Magnetic resonance tomography	31 %

Table 6.5: Frequency of pathological findings in instrumental investigations in neuroborreliosis stages II and III

This can occasionally be helpful in differential diagnosis versus e.g. a slipped disc, if only monoradicular pain symptoms are present. In addition, neurophysiological investigation techniques can be used for a prognostic evaluation of the course. Among the imaging procedures, magnetic resonance tomography (MRT) should be tried first. The computed tomogram gave a pathological finding in only 7 of 83 of our own patients investigated to date. MRT, on the other hand, revealed inflammatory changes of the spinal cord, brainstem, or white or gray matter in 13 out of 42 cases. The lesions might indicate focal parenchymatous inflammation or local vasculitis. Clinically silent signal intensifications are detectable in up to 50 % of patients with tertiary neuroborreliosis. Multiple periventricular signal intensifications are extremely rare, and so differential diagnosis against multiple sclerosis is seldom a neuroradiological concern.

As regards the value of instrumental methods for further clarification of Lyme carditis, no experience is available apart from the already described changes in the ECG. A similar situation exists for Lyme arthritis, where all that is known is that nonspecific radiological alterations of the affected joint are detectable in up to 80 % of the cases.

6.1.2. Nonspecific laboratory changes in blood, CSF, and synovial fluid

Among the nonspecific inflammation parameters (☞ Table 6.6) the ESR, CRP, and circulating immune complexes are most commonly slightly elevated in blood. Leukocytosis and elevated serum levels of IgM and the complement components C3 and C4 are rarely detectable. Comparison of seronegative and seropositive control groups revealed no disease-specific constellation of laboratory values. Circulating immune complexes are also detectable in 60 % of asymptomatic infected individuals and in other disease pictures (e.g. collagenosis). They are useful as nonspecific activity parameters, because they disappear during treatment and persist on development of secondary disease phenomena after ECM. *Borrelia*-specific antigens can be isolated from immune complexes. In a study carried out in the US this was apparently possible in 95 % of the sera investigated. No other reports are available. As evidence of additional organ manifestations, slight elevation of liver and pancreas-specific enzymes is detectable in 42 % and 32 % of the patients respectively. Fulminant hepatitis is not reported, although the transaminases can be up to 100 times the normal limit. Microhematuria associated with mild proteinuria is observed, serum creatinine and urinary substances remaining in the normal range. No elevation of creatine kinase was detectable in the Lyme myocarditis patients described in the literature, nor indeed among our own patients.

The suspicion of an inflammatory disease of the nervous system is confirmed by **analysis of the CSF**. This typically shows lymphocytic pleocytosis, though the cell count may be normal in very early forms of peripheral neurogenic damage, ACA-associated polyneuritis and previously

6.1. Lyme borreliosis

Parameter	Normal values	Mean (range)	Pathological values/ investigated patients (%)
Serum			
ESR	5-18	35 (4-68)	141/214 (66 %)
CRP (mg/dl)	< 5.0	5.7 (< 5.0-38)	17/33 (51 %)
Leukocytes	4000-11 000	7600 (3200-18 600)	14/145 (10 %)
Circulating immune complexes (µgEg/ml)	< 6 (Clq-ELISA)	6.8 (1.1-15.8)	13/30 (43 %)
	< 21 (RCR-ELISA)	12.7 (4.4-26.1)	4/30 (13 %)
SGOT (U/l)	5-20	10 (4-30)	8/158 (5 %)
SGPT (U/l)	5-23	17 (4-82)	39/158 (25 %)
γ-GT (U/l)	4-28	21 (5-353)	43/158 (27 %)
Cerebrospinal fluid			
Cell count (n/µl)	< 4	90 (2-1100)	315/330 (96 %)
Total protein (g/l)	< 0.5	1.4 (0.13-10.7)	282/330 (85 %)
Oligoclonal bands	negative		170/257 (66 %)
IgM$_{loc}$ (mg/dl)	negative	34.0 (0-250)	70/135 (52 %)
IgA$_{loc}$ (mg/dl)	negative	7.3 (0-316)	28/139 (20 %)
IgG$_{loc}$ (mg/dl)	negative	70.0 (0-985)	62/245 (25 %)
Lactate (mmol/l)	< 1.9	2.2 (0.28-5.3)	123/245 (50 %)

Table 6.6: Frequency of pathological serum and CSF findings in neuroborreliosis

treated patients. Depending on the patient population investigated, the frequency of pleocytosis is 95-100 %, in agreement with other European authors. In the United States it is distinctly lower, possibly on account of the diagnostic criteria which by European standards are inadequate. The cell count elevation is generally moderate. In further differential diagnosis the cytology is helpful. A lymphocytic cell picture is typical, which with advancing disease may contain more pronounced stimulated cell forms with dividing formations and multiple cell nuclei. Immunocytochemically, numerous activated B-lymphocytes are detectable. None of our own patients showed more than 10 % of granulocytes in the differential blood count. In half of the patients lactate is generally only slightly elevated. 85 % of patients show elevated total protein, with average values of 1.4 g/l. At the extreme, patients with chronic courses can show values up to 11.3 g/l. The elevated total protein values in neuroborreliosis are nearly always due to a disturbance of the blood-brain barrier, as confirmed by the pathological albumin ratios. Determination of this ratio is a prerequisite for calculating intrathecal immunoglobulin synthesis, which is present in 20 % (IgA), 25 % (IgG), and 52 % (IgM) of the cases. Our own data show that detection of local IgG synthesis depends on the time at which the infection has occurred, which explains the differences between the literature figures. Oligoclonal band determination detects local IgG synthesis in a distinctly higher percentage of cases because it is more sensitive. A feature that distinguishes neuroborreliosis from other infectious diseases of the CNS is the striking dominance of IgM in comparison with other immunoglobulins (IgG, IgA).

Each of the individual parameters mentioned can, to varying extents, show pathological changes in other CNS inflammations as well. A literature survey of various constellations of pathological parameters was therefore carried out with a view to establishing their predictive value.

> For the combination of lymphocytic pleocytosis with a disturbance of the blood-brain barrier, intrathecal IgG synthesis, and intrathecal synthesis of IgM and/or IgA, a specificity of 99 % and a sensitivity of 88.5 % have been cited.

According to other data the CSF syndrome comprising

- dominant intrathecal IgM synthesis
- activated IgM-containing B-lymphocytes and
- a disturbance of the blood-brain barrier

shows a specificity of 96 % and a sensitivity of 70 %. According to our own findings, although these CSF syndromes are indeed characteristic of neuroborreliosis, the dynamics of the inflammatory process mean that they are only present in patients who have been ill for 4 to 6 weeks. In the first week only a slight barrier disruption without local IgG synthesis may be detectable, with a slightly elevated cell count. At this time only a few hypersegmented granulocytes and numerous IgM-containing active B lymphocytes are detectable in the cell sediment. As the disease progresses, marked local IgM synthesis becomes detectable, with the appearance of oligoclonal bands from the third week. Milder acutely inflammatory changes and local synthesis of IgG, IgA, and IgM are typical of patients with a longer history.

The varying protein pattern can be helpful in ruling out other inflammatory diseases. Patients with neurosyphilis, for example, are characterized by an intact blood-brain barrier and a one- or two-class reaction in the absence of IgA synthesis. Neurotuberculosis shows a two-class reaction with IgA dominance, lactate invariably being conspicuously elevated. In ruling out multiple sclerosis it is useful that, in MS, non-dominant IgM synthesis occurs in only 25-50 % of the cases and IgA synthesis in 1 %. Indeed, in our own study none of the 20 MS control patients investigated showed any elevation of IgM or IgA. Moreover, the fraction of neuroborreliosis patients who show an MS CSF syndrome (cell count < 50/µl, normal total protein, and positive oligoclonal bands) can be distinguished by the additional determination of IgM and IgA. The MRZ (measles-rubella-zoster) reaction is unhelpful in the differential diagnosis because MS, tertiary neuroborreliosis, and lupus erythematosus can all give a positive finding. A CSF syndrome compatible with idiopathic polyradiculoneuritis or with root compression syndrome has never been observed among our patients. Literature reports of the occurrence of such CSF findings have not been adequately corroborated.

The findings described here emphasize the usefulness of CSF diagnostics in consolidating a tentative clinical diagnosis of neuroborreliosis. As the results of pathogen-specific diagnostics may be unavailable for a few days, or may still be negative at the first lumbar puncture, the general CSF finding is helpful in deciding on antibiotic therapy. The literature findings indicating that the majority of patients initially have a highly specific CSF syndrome cannot be confirmed. In patients with uncharacteristic CSF changes the tentative diagnosis can only be confirmed via the pathogen-specific investigation procedure, which is described in detail in Section 6.1.3.

In addition to the serum and the CSF, the **synovial fluid** can be diagnostically useful. Puncture is advisable to rule out effusions due to physical irritation in arthrosis and septic arthritis. The puncture fluid is also useful for direct and indirect pathogen diagnosis. A positive microbiological finding would then unambiguously confirm the etiopathogenesis in the individual case.

6.1.3. Microbiological diagnosis of Lyme borreliosis

Like syphilis, the human *Borrelia* infection progresses in stages and sometimes manifests itself multisystemically. The description of Lyme borreliosis as a separate clinical entity, the identification of the pathogen (☞ Fig. 6.1), and the clarification of the transmission pathway in the early eighties led to a wealth of new knowledge and discoveries in microbiological diagnostics as well.

6.1. Lyme borreliosis

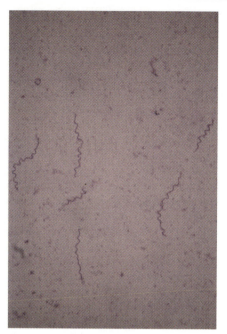

Fig. 6.1: B. burgdorferi, Giemsa stain, 1000 ×, oil-immersion objective

The variety of clinical symptoms has made Lyme borreliosis the new chameleon of medicine and raises a number of differential-diagnostic problems. On clinical suspicion the preference nowadays is for a laboratory diagnosis, which despite the considerable advances is still difficult. For diagnosis of the pathogen a number of direct and indirect test procedures are available (☞ Table 6.7).

Direct detection methods	Indirect detection methods
• Direct microscopy[2]	• Indirect hemagglutination test (IHAT)[1]
• Culture of the pathogen[2]	• Complement fixation reaction (CFR)[1]
• Polymerase chain reaction (PCR)[2]	• Enzyme-linked immunosorbent assay (ELISA)[1]
• *Borrelia*-specific antigen detection[2]	• Immunofluorescence assay (IFA)[1]
	• Full antigen immunoblot[1]
	• Recombinant immunoblot[1]
	• Serum bactericidal activity test[2]

Table 6.7: Microbiological borreliosis diagnostics: standard serological tests (1) and special or experimental test procedures (2)

Test methods

Standard serological tests (e.g. ELISA, IFA, immunoblot) for indirect detection of the pathogen are now widely used in routine diagnostics in the microbiological laboratory.

Further **special and experimental tests**, particularly microscopy, culture, and the polymerase chain reaction (PCR) for direct detection of the pathogen, but also the test for bactericidal action in serum for diagnosis of bactericidal antibodies in Lyme borreliosis, are generally confined to special laboratories. Some of these tests are still at the evaluation stage.

All these diagnostic laboratory procedures require a critical evaluation of their capabilities and must be continually assessed for their diagnostic power in everyday clinical practice. They also require further standardization in methodology and diagnostic evaluation, to ensure consistent quality in the diagnosis of Lyme borreliosis. The following sections illustrate the capabilities and limitations of modern investigation methods in borreliosis diagnostics, with an explanation and evaluation of their diagnostic status in everyday practice.

6.1.3.1. Diagnostic methods for direct pathogen detection in Lyme borreliosis

6.1.3.1.1. Direct microscopic detection

Various microscopic methods are available for examining suitable specimen materials (CSF, blood, joint puncture fluid, biopsy material, tick homogenate) for *Borrelia* (☞ Table 6.8). As the characteristic morphology of the pathogens is often obscured by fixation and staining, however, the results of conventional light microscopy are often contradictory, and inexperienced operators may find it difficult to distinguish positive findings from artifacts and non-pathogenic spirochetes. In addition to light microscopy, some laboratories use fluorescence microscopy and electron microscopy for direct detection of *Borreliae* in specimen material. As the pathogen concentration in most clinical specimens (blood, CSF, and biopsies) is very low, however, in the majority of cases direct microscopy fails to detect *Borreliae* even after enrichment of the pathogen in liquids by centrifugation. A negative microscopic finding does not in any case rule out the presence of disease, and so the use of microscopy is restricted to selected cases or to scientific investigations. Only dark-field and phase-contract microscopy have found a firm place in experimental work and in the diagnosis of high microbial counts in cultures.

6.1.3.1.2. Detection of the pathogen by culture

The *Borrelia* infection enters via the skin as the portal of entry, and only subsequently is the pathogen carried via the blood to various other target organs, particularly to the central nervous system and the joints. The literature contains reports of successful *Borrelia* culture from practically all clinically relevant materials (puncture fluids, blood, CSF, biopsy material). *Borreliae* are generally extremely demanding bacteria with a long generation time (7-20 hours), and must be cultured in nutrient-rich liquid media supplemented with bovine albumin. Modified Barbour-Stoenner-Kelly (BSK) medium has proved particularly suitable (☞ Section 2.1.3.). In case of contaminated specimen material the liquid culture can additionally be supplemented with a combination of antibiotics to prevent any overgrowth with rapidly growing concomitant flora. Owing to the long generation time the cultures must be incubated for at least 5 weeks at 30-33°C, and require subculturing at least once weekly and dark-field microscopy to check for possible growth. Many authors also perform a PCR control test (☞ Section 6.1.3.1.4.) on cultures showing no microscopic signs of overgrowth, so as not to overlook low microbial counts. The procedure for culturing *Borreliae* is shown in Fig. 6.2.

Method	Stain	Material
Light microscopy	Giemsa stain, carbol fuchsin stain, silver stains	Skin biopsies, whole blood, CSF, synovial biopsy, culture material
Dark-field microscopy, Phase-contrast microscopy	Native specimen	Tick homogenate, culture material, biopsy material
Electron microscopy		Skin biopsies, whole blood, CSF, synovial biopsy, culture material
Immunofluorescence microscopy	Staining with fluorescein-labeled specific antibodies	Blood CSF, puncture fluid, tick homogenate, culture material

Tab. 6.8: Microscopic methods for direct detection of *B. burgdorferi* s.l.

6.1. Lyme borreliosis

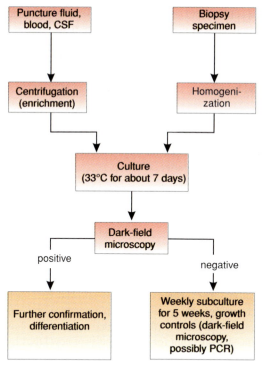

Fig. 6.2: Procedure for culturing of *Borreliae*

Blood, puncture fluid, samples of cerebrospinal fluid, and biopsy material obtained under sterile conditions can be used for the culture, and it is best to transfer them directly into culture tubes containing modified BSK medium. The blood, puncture fluid, and cerebrospinal fluid can first be concentrated by centrifugation. The decisive factors for successful culture are pathogen density and sterile sampling, but also rapid transport and optimal working up of the samples. The nature of the material and the duration of the infection (disease stage) are also important.

Specimens taken from patients in the early stages of disease are more likely to be successful than those from patients in the later stages or those who have already been given antibiotic treatment. Skin biopsies, particularly from the region of the tick bite, have a moderate success rate of about 60 %, but this is substantially higher in the presence of erythema migrans or acrodermatitis chronica atrophicans (ACA) (about 80-90 %). *Borrelia* can sometimes be cultured from biopsy material months after the skin lesion has healed up, but a substantially lower percentage of positive results is obtained from cultures made using blood (1-3 %), cerebrospinal fluid (5-20 %), or puncture fluid.

Summarizing, the culture of *Borreliae* remains expensive and time-consuming, and has a low success rate, particularly in the diagnostically difficult later stages of the disease. Since culture requires much experience, identification in this way will generally continue to be limited to specialist laboratories. However, a positive culture can definitively confirm the diagnosis of Lyme borreliosis and is therefore very valuable, particularly in problem patients. If the growth of a culture is to be attempted, arrangements with the microbiology laboratory must be made in advance and care must be taken to ensure optimal transport of the specimen in a suitable medium.

6.1.3.1.3. Antibiotic sensitivity testing of *Borrelia burgdorferi* s.l.

In principle it is possible to test the sensitivity of *B. burgdorferi* s.l. isolates to antibiotics. Modified BSK medium supplemented with defined concentrations of the substance to be tested can be used to determine the minimal inhibitory concentration (MIC).

> The MIC is defined as the lowest concentration of an antibiotic which completely inhibits multiplication of the microorganisms.

The initial microbial concentration is about 10^5/ml and the culture time is about 72-96 h at 33°C. Because of the long generation time of *Borreliae*, the detection of an antibiotic effect requires at least 24 h (E. coli: approx. 4 h). The minimal inhibitory concentration recorded is the lowest antibiotic concentration which results in no *Borreliae* being visible under a dark-field microscope after a maximum of 72-96 h. In addition to the sensitivity and the long generation time of the pathogen, individual differences in antibiotic degradation rates during the long culture periods involved in the resistance determination represent a problem. However, culture of the pathogen only succeeds in a fraction of the cases diagnosed clinically, so the methods mentioned are used largely in experimental studies and rarely in routine microbiological work.

Up to now the choice of the antibiotic was based essentially on empirical data from therapeutic studies in patients with Lyme borreliosis and on information about the pharmacological profiles of the substances (MIC, levels in plasma and cerebrospinal fluid). Table 6.9 shows the most effective antibiotics against *B. burgdorferi* s.l. in vitro.

Antibiotic	MIC (mg/l)	
	MIC range	MIC 90
Penicillin G	0.50-8.0	4.0
Amoxicillin	0.25-1.0	0.50
Mezlocillin	0.25-1.0	0.50
Ceftriaxone	0.03-0.25	0.06
Cefotaxime	0.06-0.25	0.12
Ceftazidime	0.12-0.25	0.12
Cefmenoxime	0.03-0.25	0.12
Cefuroxime	0.12-0.50	0.25
Cefixime	0.12-0.50	0.25
Azithromycin	0.015-0.03	0.015
Clarithromycin	0.015-0.06	0.015
Erythromycin	0.03-0.12	0.06
Roxithromycin	0.015-0.12	0.03
Tetracycline HCl	0.25-2.0	1.0
Doxycycline	0.12-1.0	0.50
Minocycline	0.12-1.0	0.50
Imipenem	0.06-1.0	0.25

Table 6.9: In-vitro efficacy of antibiotics against *B. burgdorferi* s.l. (according to Preac-Mursic 1992). The MIC (minimal inhibitory concentration) 90 is the lowest concentration of an antimicrobial substance which inhibits the growth of at least 90 % of the strains tested

6.1.3.1.4. Direct detection with the aid of the polymerase chain reaction

Principle

Direct microscopy and culture quickly reach their limits in the detection of pathogens which are difficult to culture. The introduction of the PCR allows a direct highly specific and very sensitive detection of fragments of the genetic material (DNA) of such microorganisms in the specimen material. The test is carried out by isolating the DNA present in the specimen and amplifying specific target genetic sequences of the pathogen (☞ Fig. 6.3).

The reaction is based on cyclic replication (amplification) of these DNA sequences *in vitro* after the addition of:

- an enzyme which synthesizes DNA (thermally stable DNA polymerase)
- a sequence-specific oligonucleotide (primer) as a reaction starter, and
- the four nucleic acid building blocks (deoxyribonucleoside triphosphates, dNTPs)

All three components are added to the reaction mixture in excess. The reaction is started by separating the DNA in the specimens into single strands by heating to 90-94°C (thermal denaturation). The primers are then allowed to attach themselves by lowering the temperature (annealing). The short double-stranded region serves as the starting point for the synthesis of new DNA by the DNA polymerase, and the dNTPs are inserted at an optimal temperature of 70-72°C (elongation). The polymerase must be thermally stable if it is to continue to function despite the cyclic temperature changes. The cycle of denaturation, annealing, and elongation is repeated 30 to 50 times (☞ Fig. 6.3). The prerequisite for the procedure is the availability of a pair of primers which are complementary to, and flank, the complementary DNA strands of the target sequence. Under optimal conditions exponential multiplication of the specific synthesis products takes place, making about 10^8-10^{10} copies. A modification of the method can be used to increase its sensitivity and specificity still further: a further targeted PCR is carried out on the PCR product already obtained, using a primer whose recognition sequences are enclosed within the gene section already amplified (nested PCR). This produces a very large number (10^{12}-10^{13}) of DNA copies of the target sequence. These should later be analyzed further to establish their specificity, using techniques such as hybridization with specific gene probes, restriction-endonuclease analysis, or DNA sequencing. To some extent further genotyping of the pathogen can be carried out, with assignment to one of the three species of *Borrelia* pathogenic in humans (*B. burgdorferi* s.s., *B. garinii, B. afzelii*) using the amplified DNA.

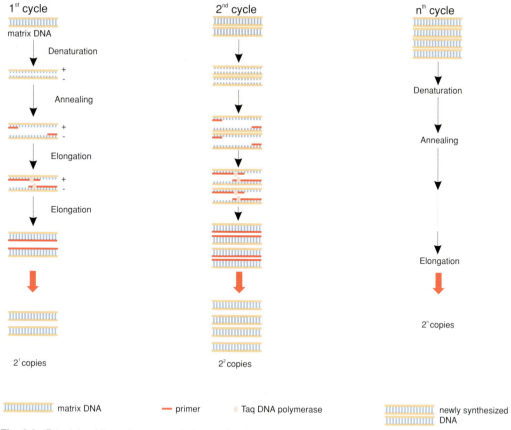

Fig. 6.3: Principle of the polymerase chain reaction (schematic)

Diagnostic value

The sensitivity of the *Borreliae*, their long generation time, and the often low microbial count in clinical specimens suggest that PCR would be a particularly promising method for the diagnosis of *B. burgdorferi* infection. The speed with which the results are obtained, within 12 to 24 h, is another advantage. Many laboratories have therefore attempted to use the methodologically difficult specific DNA detection for *B. burgdorferi* s.l. as a diagnostic method. Suitable starting materials are in particular cerebrospinal fluid or arthrocentesis material, only exceptionally blood or urine. The limit of detection of the method varies depending on the investigator and the technique used, the literature citing values of 0.002 to 0.1 pg of purified *B. burgdorferi* DNA. This corresponds to a sensitivity of 2 to 100 *Borreliae* in the specimen. The principal target sequences used for *B. burgdorferi* s.l.
are specific plasmid-encoded gene sequences for the outer surface proteins A and B (OspA and OspB) and chromosomal gene sequences (flagellin, 16S-RNA gene, p66/Oms66 gene). Genetic cross-reactivity with other *Borrelia* species has been reported only in rare cases.

However, the PCR results in the diagnosis of *B. burgdorferi* infection obtained by different workers are extremely contradictory, and the results of recent studies show substantial variability in sensitivity of the method. It also seems to be necessary to carry out several analyses of the specimens using different primers, because a single sample may give a positive PCR result with one pair of primers and a negative result with another. In addition, the material processing technique and the methodology can result in both false positive results due to DNA contamination and false negative results due to inhibitors (e.g. heparin or hemoglobin) in the specimen.

Furthermore, since so far neither the conditions of specimen collection, transport, and working up, nor the method have been standardized, PCR results obtained in different laboratories are still not comparable. This fact, along with the substantial costs of apparatus and personnel, has delayed more widespread use of the method as a routine diagnostic tool. So far the PCR must be classified as a supplementary method, and not a substitute for an established test procedure. It is therefore desirable to evaluate its results in the light of results obtained with other microbiological test procedures. The indication for a PCR test for *Borrelia* should accordingly continue to be limited to selected cases difficult to identify by differential diagnostics, and the test should only be carried out by selected laboratories. Preference should also be given to clinically relevant materials such as cerebrospinal fluid or joint puncture fluid. It is not possible to draw any conclusions about the viability and infectivity of the pathogen on the basis of a positive PCR result.

At present the PCR technique plays a subordinate role in Lyme borreliosis diagnostics, and the determination of its value in *Borrelia* diagnosis and the development of clear guidelines for its use in diagnostic laboratories remain the subjects of future work.

6.1.3.1.5. Detection of Borrelia-specific antigens in clinical specimens

Infection of a macroorganism with a pathogen is followed by the release of immunogenic antigenic determinants which, depending on the point of entry, may circulate in the blood or body fluids or sometimes accumulate in the tissue. Detection of the antigens as a diagnostic method is already in practical use in a large number of infectious diseases. The first evidence for the possible relevance of antigen detection in specimen material in the diagnosis of Lyme borreliosis was obtained from studies in *Borrelia*-infected hamsters and mice. Antigens to the pathogen were detected in the animals' urine by the ELISA technique using specific monoclonal antibodies. Further studies demonstrated the presence of specific antigens in clinically relevant specimens from Lyme borreliosis patients. The outer surface proteins, in particular the OspA of *B. burgdorferi* s.l., were detected most often. This approach seems most promising as a diagnostic test for neuroborreliosis in cerebrospinal fluid. As well as having diagnostic relevance, detection of antigens in the cerebrospinal fluid could become important for monitoring the course of the disease during treatment: studies have shown a fall of the antigen concentration measured to below the limit of detection within 2-6 weeks of successful treatment in previously antigen-positive neuroborreliosis patients. However, the prerequisite is the availability of highly sensitive test systems which can reliably detect even the low antigen concentrations in *Borrelia*-infected patients in various stages of the disease. The known antigenic heterogeneity of different European *Borrelia* species also needs to be taken into account in the choice of the specific antibodies used. The diagnostic significance of these test methods still needs to be demonstrated experimentally in clinical studies.

6.1.3.1.6. Methods of differentiating species

So far, three genospecies of the *B. burgdorferi* s.l. complex pathogenic in humans have been identified in Europe on the basis of their phenotypic and genotypic properties (*B. burgdorferi* s.s., *B. garinii*, *B. afzelii*), and the possibility of them having differing organotropism has been discussed. Direct detection of *Borrelia* in culture therefore necessitates further microbiological differentiation of the organisms to identify the species (☞ Table 6.10).

Typing procedures for B. burgdorferi s.l.
• 5S-rDNA sequence analysis
• Analysis of the macrorestriction pattern of genomic DNA by pulsed-field gel electrophoresis (PFGE) after enzymatic digestion with low-cleavage-rate restriction endonucleases
• OspA/OspC serotyping using monoclonal antibodies

Table 6.10: Typing procedures for *B. burgdorferi* s.l.

One method of differentiation is an analysis of the macrorestriction pattern of genomic DNA of corresponding isolates by pulsed-field gel electrophoresis (PFGE) after enzymatic digestion with rare cutting restriction enzymes (endonucleases).

However, the actual genetic classification is carried out on the basis of sequence analyses of species-specific ribosomal gene sections. It is also possible to carry out a phenotypic classification of isolates into serotypes by using monoclonal antibodies to the heterogeneous outer surface proteins OspA and OspC of *B. burgdorferi* s.l. The current methods of phenotypic and genotypic species differentiation of *Borrelia burgdorferi* s.l. are summarized in Table 6.10. For further details see the descriptions in Section 2.1.4. Direct detection of the pathogen by PCR also permits a more detailed analysis of the amplified target sequence, with classification into the known species of *Borrelia* (see Section 6.1.3.1.4.). However, the use of any of the genetic techniques requires a substantial outlay on apparatus and personnel, and consequently these techniques are still largely restricted to molecular biology research laboratories.

6.1.3.2. Indirect detection of the pathogen (serological detection of antibodies)

Despite the substantial advances in our knowledge of properties of the pathogen and the many new diagnostic methods, serological detection of antibodies remains the method of choice in Lyme borreliosis diagnostics because of its reliability and the simplicity of specimen collection. During the methodological development of test systems and of the interpretation of results it was possible to make some use of experience with the diagnosis of treponematoses, particularly syphilis. At the same time, however, it must be said that serological diagnosis of Lyme borreliosis is still far from reaching similar high quality of standardization in the test procedure and interpretation of the findings, since diagnostic tools do not require registration and a wide range of commercial tests of differing quality is on the market. Together with the long-established classical methods of serological detection such as the indirect immunofluorescence assay (IFA), the complement-fixation reaction (CFR), and the indirect hemagglutination test (IHAT), the introduction of ELISA and the immunoblot using constantly improving antigen products makes available a whole series of tested techniques for serological diagnostics. It is sensible to combine highly sensitive screening methods with very specific confirmatory tests. The diagnostic value in specific cases is to some extent influenced by the individual course of the infection and by the antibody response, i.e. by the patient's immunological status. Experience in carrying out serological tests and in the interpretation of the results also plays an important role in the quality and reproducibility of diagnostic tests for borreliosis in the microbiological laboratory.

6.1.3.2.1. Stage-dependent antibody kinetics in Lyme borreliosis

Knowledge of the temporal course of the antibody response to the immunodominant antigens of the pathogen is very useful in the evaluation of serological findings. The antigenic specificities of the membrane proteins and flagellin from *B. burgdorferi* s.l. have been the subjects of extensive investigations. By contrast, there is still little definite information about the structure and immunological significance of the lipid and carbohydrate components.

Specific antibodies against *Borrelia* antigens can usually be detected 3-6 weeks after the infection has taken place. The formation of IgM antibodies usually precedes that of IgG antibodies, but in individual cases IgM production may be delayed or even absent altogether. The primary immune response to early infections by both classes of immunoglobulin is only directed against a few antigens, in particular against components of flagellin (p41) and the outer surface protein OspC of *B. burgdorferi* s.l. OspC is of particular diagnostic relevance because of its pathogen specificity. All the same, a substantial proportion of false negatives should be expected in the early stages of Lyme borreliosis, as some patients build up a significant antibody titer only very slowly. Seroprevalence studies show a serologically detectable antibody response in 20 to 80 % of patients with local infections (stage I), depending on the test method and test criteria used.

Stage	Proportion of seropositive patients in %	IgM response in %	IgG response in %
I	20-80	up to 90	up to 70
II	50-90	30-80	65-100
III	95-100	5-48	100

Table 6.11: Stage dependence of the antibody pattern in Lyme borreliosis patients. The percentages given are guideline figures, and can vary according to the test system and the *B. burgdorferi* s.l. isolate used for antigen preparation

IgM antibodies can be detected in up to 90 % of seropositive patients, but a corresponding IgG response is only present in up to 70 % of the cases. The number of seropositive patients increases as the *Borrelia* infection progresses (stage II and III) (☞ Table 6.11).

IgG-type antibodies directed against a number of *Borrelia* antigens are characteristic of the acute disseminated and chronic organ manifestations (stages II and III of Lyme borreliosis). Antibodies against specific antigens such as the p83/100 protein, BmpA (p39), the internal fragment of flagellin (p41i), and p18 are of particularly high diagnostic significance. In contrast, antibodies against the outer surface protein OpsA, which is also very specific, are rare because of a change in antigen presentation by the pathogen from OspA to OspC in the human host (see Section 2.1.4.).

An important prerequisite for serological detection of antibodies is a normal immune status and the ability of the patient to produce antibodies (☞ Table 6.12).

The possibility of rare cases of seronegative Lyme borreliosis should be borne in mind in patients with stubborn disease courses with clinically unambiguous symptoms. Direct detection of the pathogen should always be considered if Lyme borreliosis is suspected in immunosuppressed patients or when unclear serological findings are repeatedly obtained.

False negative *Borrelia* serology	False positive *Borrelia* serology
• Low antibody titer in early stages of the disease (sensitivity gap)	• Cross reactions in infections due to other pathogens: *viruses:* CMV, EBV, other herpes viruses *bacteria:* spirochetes, Enterobacteriaceae, *Neisseria*, pneumococci etc.
• Antigenic heterogeneity of the pathogen: certain specific antigens formed are not detected by the test system (sensitivity gap)	• Diseases of the autoimmune and rheumatic type
• Immunosuppression, HIV	
• False negative IgM test due to a high specific IgG titer (negative immunological feedback)	

Table 6.12: Possible causes of false positive and false negative reactions in borreliosis serology

6.1.3.2.2. Serological tests in Lyme borreliosis diagnostics

Indirect hemagglutination test (IHAT)

The IHAT is a classical economic serological technique used for the diagnosis of many infectious diseases. It has a high sample throughput, permitting its use in screening. Antibody detection in Lyme borreliosis is carried out using sheep erythrocytes loaded with a mixture of antigens made from *Borrelia* ultrasonicate and untreated control erythrocytes. The test system detects both IgG and IgM antibodies. The test delivers qualitative and quantitative information and may have adequate sensitivity, depending on the antigen mixture used, but it must be followed by a class- and antigen-specific analysis of the immunoglobulins using a suitable method of confirmation (immunoblot) for further differentiation of the immune response and because of the low specificity. The introduction of modern ELISAs with higher sensitivity and specificity into borreliosis diagnostics has reduced the importance of the IHAT.

Complement-fixation reaction (CFR)

The reaction is used to detect complement-activating antibodies (IgM and IgG), but because of its low sensitivity and specificity in the diagnosis of borreliosis it is no longer the procedure of first choice.

Indirect Immunofluorescence assay (IFA)

The IFA is carried out by washing freshly cultured *Borreliae* in the exponential growth phase, fixing them to microscope slides with acetone or methanol, and covering the slides with test sera. The binding of specific antibodies can be visualized under a fluorescence microscope by using fluorescein-isothiocyanate-labeled polyvalent or class-specific antihuman antibodies (for IgG and IgM) (☞ Fig. 6.4).

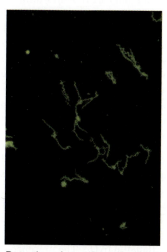

Fig. 6.4: Detection of specific antibodies to *B. burgdorferi* s.l. in the immunofluorescence test (460 nm, 1000 ×, oil-immersion objective)

The IFA can thus be used both as a screening test and also to quantify the antibody response in cerebrospinal fluid and serum. Historically, it was one of the first serological tests developed for the diagnosis of Lyme borreliosis. Since pure cultures of individual strains are used in the majority of IFAs, the known antigenic variability of the different species of the *B. burgdorferi* s.l. complex mean that the sensitivity and specificity of the test are substantially dependent on the isolate used and on the nature of the patient's antibodies. False positive reactions for IgM antibodies are sometimes obtained in untreated serum samples, usually as a result of a positive rheumatoid factor. Nonspecific cross reactions are also possible, particularly after infections with other spirochetes (see Table 6.12). The IFA plays an increasingly subordinate role in *Borrelia* diagnostics, and is used mainly as a reserve test to answer special questions (determination of the CSF-serum index) or when the confirmatory test (immunoblot) has given an ambiguous result with a strong suspicion of a nonspecific reaction.

■ ELISA

The general principle of solid-phase ELISA is based on the detection of specific antibodies after binding to antigen-coated microtiter plates, using enzyme-labeled antihuman IgG or IgM antibodies (sandwich principle, ☞ Fig. 6.5a).

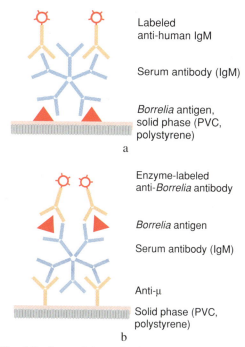

Fig. 6.5a+b: **a**: Schematic diagram of solid-phase IgM ELISA. **b**: Functional principle of an anti-µ test system

The positive reaction obtained after addition of the substrate can then be measured photometrically. The nature and the quality of the antigen products used are decisive for diagnostic standardization. In addition to the use of ultrasonic extracts of *B. burgdorferi* s.l., which have a low level of standardization, attempts have been made to increase the specificity of the test system without losing sensitivity by concentrating specific antigens such as OspC using detergent extraction, by using purified flagellin (selective ELISA), or by using recombinant antigens (recombinant ELISA). The use of a combination of various antigenic determinants avoids diagnostic gaps and enables *Borrelia*-specific antibodies from early and late stages of the immune response to be recognized. Recombinant antigen products should allow for the marked heterogeneity of the species-specific protein pattern and as far as possible should cover all known *Borrelia* species. Depending on the manufacturer, it may be possible to carry out qualitative detection of specific antibodies and to obtain quantitative information on the course of infection by converting the optical density measurements into test-specific units, analogously to the course of the titers in IFA, though ELISA has the advantage of substantially higher precision. The factors which interfere with the test are essentially the same as in IFA. Preabsorption of the specimen is therefore necessary. Another possibility for the detection of specific IgM antibodies is capture-ELISA using solid-phase antihuman antibodies (☞ Fig. 6.5b).

Because of its relatively good specificity and high sensitivity, ELISA is now the method of choice in the first step of the serological borreliosis diagnostics (screening test).

Immunoblot technique for the serological antibody detection in borreliosis diagnostics

The Western-blot technique

The Western-blot technique is based on the transfer of proteins already separated by polyacrylamide gel electrophoresis to a nitrocellulose or polyvinyl difluoride (PVDF) membrane. Hydrophobic interactions cause the proteins to remain fixed to the membrane, and they can be stored in this form. The antigen products used play a decisive role as far as quality is concerned. The technique offers a serological test system of high sensitivity and specificity. One particular advantage of the method is that it can reliably identify a large number of antigen-specific antibodies. The test is carried out by incubating antigen-treated blot strips with the patient's serum (immunoblot). When specific antibodies bind to the proteins, they can be identified as colored bands in a second step by using enzyme-labeled antihuman antibodies in a manner similar to the sandwich principle in ELISA. Each band corresponds to an antibody reaction with the underlying antigen fraction. However, unlike in the ELISA technique, this method does not just detect the presence of antibodies. Instead, the nature and number of bands in an immunoblot permits exact class- and antigen-specific analysis of the antibody pattern formed.

In diagnosis of borreliosis it is necessary to distinguish between a whole-cell-antigen immunoblot and a recombinant immunoblot (☞ Fig. 6.6):

■ Whole-cell-antigen immunoblot

The starting material used for the whole-cell-antigen immunoblot are *Borrelia*-ultrasonicate extracts obtained from pure cultures of strains of *Borrelia* during the exponential phase of growth. The advantage of the method is that all naturally occurring antigens of the strain are applied and are available for the antibody detection. However, in addition to highly specific antigens numerous less specific or nonspecific antigens are present (☞ Table 6.13), and they can react with antibodies from the patient (IgM and/or IgG).

In addition, reliable identification and correct weighting of the bands are decisive for the quality of the diagnosis. A finding of specific IgM antibodies in the whole-cell-antigen immunoblot is regarded as particularly well established if two of the following three bands are detected: OspC, BmpA (p39) and flagellin (p41). The presence of several of the following bands is regarded as particularly diagnostically informative in the detection of specific IgG antibodies: p18, OspC, OspA, BmpA (p39), flagellin (p41), Oms 66 (p66), and p83/100.

One diagnostic difficulty is that the immunodominant antigens of the three *Borrelia* species pathogenic in humans which are so far known in Europe show a certain amount of variability. Serological studies relating to this factor have shown that not all strains of *Borrelia* are equally suitable for preparation of the antigen products for whole-cell-antigen immunoblot diagnostics.

6.1. Lyme borreliosis

Protein	Stage-dependence of the marker	Specificity	Cross-reactions
p83/100	late phase	+++	(+)
p75	late phase	-	+
Oms66 (p66)	late phase	+	++
p41 (flagellin)	early/late phase	+	++
BmpA (p39)	late phase	++	(+)
OspA	late phase	+	(+)
OspC	early/late phase	+++	(+)
p41 internal	early/late phase	++	+
p21	early/late phase	-	++
p18	late phase	++	(+)

Table 6.13: Cross reactivity and specificity on the example of various *Borrelia* antigens after separation of the protein fractions in SDS gel.
Specificity: - none, + moderate, ++ good, +++ high; *Cross reactions*: (+) possible, + rare, ++ frequent; *Early phase*: stage I; *Late phase*: stages II and III

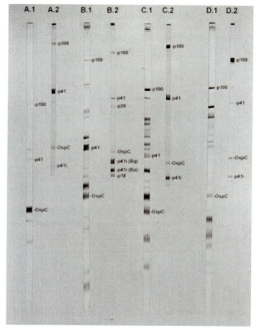

Fig. 6.6: Serological reactions of various patient sera with *Borrelia*-specific proteins in whole-cell-antigen and recombinant immunoblot:
A: erythema migrans, B: neuroborreliosis, C: Lyme arthritis, D: acrodermatitis chronica atrophicans. A.1, B.1, C.1, D.1: complete antigen immunoblot (IgG) with B. afzelii antigen; A.2, B.2, C.2, D.2: recombinant immunoblot (IgG)
Borrelia-specific proteins: p83/100, BmpA/p39, flagellin (p41), OspC, internal fragment of flagellin from B. garinii and B. afzelii (p41i [Bg] and p41i [Ba]), p18

■ Recombinant immunoblot

The recombinant immunoblot technique makes use of defined, highly purified, *Borrelia* proteins produced by genetic engineering which are transferred to the blot membrane after separation by gel electrophoresis. In positive tests there is a reaction between the patient's antibodies (IgM and/or IgG) and a few immunodominant predominantly *Borrelia*-specific antigens [p83/100, flagellin, and internal fragment (p41, p41 internal), BmpA/p39, OspA, OspC, and p18].

It is advantageous to use different antigen preparations from different *Borrelia* species on a single blot, so that antibodies to specific antigenic determinants of all three pathogens responsible for human borreliosis *(B. burgdorferi* s.s., *B. garinii, B. afzelii)* can be detected in a single test. One disadvantage of these tests up to now has been their substantial cost and their slightly lower sensitivity. The diagnostic evaluation of recombinant immunoblot tests is based on the criteria cited above, but in individual cases it depends on the manufacturer and batch as well as on the antigen products used.

■ Value of the immunoblot test in serological borreliosis diagnostics

The immunoblot technique, sometimes with the use of recombinant antigens, makes available confirmatory tests of high specificity and sensitivity. It is possible to allow for the pronounced antigenic heterogeneity of *B. burgdorferi* s.l. by using recombinant antigens or ultrasonicate extracts from different *Borrelia* species. In addition, recombinant proteins include conserved amino-acid sequences which are recognized by antibodies to antigens from all three species pathogenic in humans. When it is carried out carefully, the immunoblot can fairly reliably distinguish between antibody responses to specific and nonspecific proteins. Further standardization of the manufacture, procedure, and evaluation is desirable.

Serum bactericidal activity test

This diagnostic system permits a patient's serum to be tested after a *Borrelia* infection to establish whether protective antibodies have formed which are able, in the presence of complement, to kill the various strains of *Borrelia* used in the test. Only those strains of *Borrelia* which are able to multiply in normal serum lacking specific antigens are suitable for use in the test. These *serum resistant strains* are then incubated with the patient's serum. If bactericidal antibodies are present, they will act together with complement to kill the *Borrelia*. In the absence of appropriate antibodies the bacteria remain able to multiply. The great majority of serum-resistant strains belong to the species *B. afzelii*. The corresponding bactericidal antibodies cannot usually be detected until the late stages of Lyme borreliosis. The test is therefore mainly suitable for diagnosing chronic manifestations of borreliosis. There are also conceivable applications in confirmation of adequate immunological protection by protective antibodies after carrying out inoculation against Lyme borreliosis. The question of the definitive indication and power of this diagnostic system is the subject of current studies.

6.1.3.3. Rational standard serological diagnostics and interpretation of findings in Lyme borreliosis

Combinations of tests for standard diagnostics

In recent years there have been many studies concerned with the improvement and standardization of serological diagnostics in Lyme borreliosis. Because of the nature of serological test methods it is usually impossible to combine absolute specificity with optimal sensitivity, and since this is the objective, it is often necessary to use a combination of very sensitive screening tests with highly specific confirmatory tests to carry out serological diagnostics which are both meticulous and economic. The improved selection of specific antigens has made it possible to replace the earlier system of diagnosis in three steps (IHAT, IFA/ELISA, immunoblot) by a two-step protocol (ELISA, immunoblot). Our own experience also shows that a combination of a screening test (ELISA) with a confirmatory test (whole-cell-antigen immunoblot, recombinant immunoblot) is in most cases sufficient for assessing Lyme borreliosis infection status. The use of other test combinations increases the risk of false results by reducing the sensitivity and specificity.

Rational stepwise diagnostics

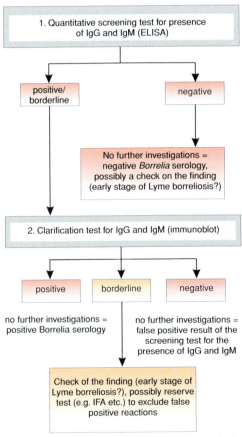

Fig. 6.7: Two-step scheme for the serological *Borrelia* diagnostics

The standard rational stepwise serological procedure for Lyme borreliosis is summarized in Fig. 6.7, and the route to follow is described briefly below:

- If the screening test is negative it is not usual to carry out any more detailed investigations and the borreliosis serology is reported as negative. However, it is not possible to exclude a *Borrelia* infection because seronegative courses are common in the early stages of the disease, and a serological control should be carried out after 2-3 weeks if clinical suspicion remains
- If, on the other hand, the screening test is positive, it is sensible to carry out further clarification with a confirmatory test. In addition to the whole-cell-antigen immunoblot, recombinant immunoblots are now available for the different *Borrelia* species. In many cases a confirmatory test carried out after a positive or borderline screening test is negative, and from a serological viewpoint borreliosis is not detectable or at most consistent with stage I or II of the disease. Once again it is sensible to carry out a serological course control if a clinical suspicion remains. If the follow-up test is positive for antibodies (IgM and IgG) against specific antigens of *B. burgdorferi* s.l., indicating seroconversion, **infection with the pathogen can be regarded as established**.
- In individual cases if the confirmatory test gives a borderline result and a nonspecific reaction is suspected an additional reserve test (e.g. IFT) should be used as a decision aid, to avoid false positive results.
- If, however, a borderline or positive screening test is supported by a confirmatory test, this fulfills the criteria for positive *Borrelia* serology. For a positive *Borrelia* serology to be qualitatively meaningful it is necessary to state which *Borrelia*-specific antigens were recognized by corresponding antibodies in the patient's serum. This is the only way to answer the question of the compatibility of the serological finding with the disease picture, i.e. with early or late stages of the disease.

Interpretation of serological findings

For a correct interpretation of the serological findings the investigator must consider a whole series of questions and facts in the evaluation of the test results. The first point to establish is whether the laboratory findings provide proof that infection has occurred. If the serological findings permit, the laboratory must carry out an analysis of the probability of a recent infection having occurred, or whether infection can be unambiguously demonstrated by proof of seroconversion. Finally, it is necessary to clarify whether the findings obtained suggest an early or a chronic stage of Lyme borreliosis. Compatibility of the serological findings with the clinical diagnosis (EM, ACA, etc.), if stated, should also be discussed.

Infection with the pathogen has taken place if antibodies to *Borrelia*-specific antigens can be identified with certainty. Further details of the time of infection can be given if antibodies (IgM/IgG) to antigens of the early phase of infection [flagellin and internal fragment (p41, p41i), OspC] suggest a relatively recent infection or if IgG seroconversion not present at a preceding examination can be demonstrated. A wide range of bands and antibodies to antigens of a later phase of infection (p83/100, p75, Oms66/p66, OspA, BmpA/p39, p18) permit the conclusion that the infection (whether symptomatic or asymptomatic) took place a fairly long time in the past. The following casuistics are intended to clarify these points.

Case 1

Multifocal erythema migrans (stage II)

About 3 weeks after a tick bite the female patient developed reddening of the skin taking the form of erythema migrans on the left thigh. At first no further investigations nor medicinal treatment were carried out. Further circumscribed erythematous foci distributed over the entire skin developed in the course of a week (multifocal erythema migrans). In the borreliosis diagnostics ordered because of the typical course both ELISA (ENZYGNOST BORRELIOSIS, Dade Behring) and recombinant immunoblot (BAG-BORRELIA-Blot, BAG) gave a positive finding for specific IgM antibodies. Oral treatment with doxycycline was started and led to a rapid improvement in the complaints. A control serological examination carried out after another 4 weeks showed seroconversion, specific IgG antibodies being detected as well.

Serology

Serology date	IgG[1]	IgM[1]	IgG[2]	IgM[2]
08.14.97	-	+	-	p41, OspC
09.10.97	72 U	+	p100, p41, p39, OspC	p41, OspC

[1] = ELISA, [2] = Immunoblot

Interpretation of the serological findings

Initially serology detected IgM antibodies to antigens (p41, OspC) which occur in the early stages of borreliosis. In the subsequent examination IgG antibodies to specific *Borrelia* antibodies were detected. The serological findings, with the detection of seroconversion, suggest infection with *B. burgdorferi* s.l. The test result is compatible with the clinical diagnosis of multifocal erythema migrans as an expression of a disseminated cutaneous form of Lyme borreliosis (stage II).

Case 2

Lyme arthritis (stage III)

The male patient had been suffering for 3 years from recurrent effusions in the knee joint of unclear origin. He remembered having had tick bites. A number of symptomatic treatments were tried, but without success. The serological test finally carried out to exclude the possibility of borreliosis gave a positive finding for specific IgG antibodies in the ELISA (ENZYGNOST BORRELIOSIS, Dade Behring) and recombinant immunoblot (BAG-BORRELIA-Blot, BAG), while the finding for IgM was negative.

3 weeks of intravenous treatment with ceftriaxone was started, and this led within a month to regression of the complaints and eventually to a complete cure.

Serology

- ELISA IgG: 540 U
- ELISA IgM: -
- Recombinant immunoblot IgG: p83/100, p39, p18
- Recombinant immunoblot IgM: -

Interpretation of the serological findings

The serological findings suggest infection with *B. burgdorferi* s.l. IgG antibodies to specific antigens of the late phase of infection (p100, p39, p18) were detected. Specific IgM antibodies were not detected. The results of the tests, when viewed together with clinical information (arthritis in the knee) are compatible with a chronic organ manifestation of Lyme borreliosis (stage III).

Case 3

Lyme arthritis (stage III)

The female patient was admitted to hospital for synovectomy following 8 months of monoarthritis with recurrent effusions in the right knee. The preoperative laboratory diagnostics showed positive borreliosis serology for IgG and IgM in the ELISA (ENZYGNOST BORRELIOSIS, Dade Behring) and the recombinant immunoblot (BAG-BORRELIA-Blot, BAG). The patient reported erythema on the left side of the neck 10 months earlier following a tick bite. 14 days of intravenous treatment with ceftriaxone led to regression of the complaints over several weeks.

Serology

- ELISA IgG: 500 U
- ELISA IgM: +
- Recombinant immunoblot IgG: p83/100, p41, OspC, p41i
- Recombinant immunoblot IgM: p100, p41, OspC, p41i

Interpretation of the serological findings

The serological findings suggested infection with *B. burgdorferi* s.l. Both IgM and IgG antibodies to specific *Borrelia* antigens were detected. From the serological viewpoint the test result is compatible with both an acute organ manifestation (stage II) and a persistent infection (stage III). In the light of the clinical information (arthritis in the knee) the finding suggests a chronic organ manifestation (stage III) of Lyme borreliosis.

Case 4

Clinical information

45-year-old woman, no other clinical information.

Serology

- ELISA IgG: 50 U
- ELISA IgM: -
- Recombinant immunoblot IgG: p83/100, p41, p41i
- Recombinant immunoblot IgM: -

■ Interpretation of the serological findings

On the basis of the serological findings it can be stated that infection with *B. burgdorferi* s.l. had occurred. IgG antibodies to *Borrelia*-specific antigens of the late phase of infection were detected (ELISA [ENZYGNOST BORRELIOSIS, Dade Behring], recombinant immunoblot [BAG-BORRELIA-Blot, BAG]). In the absence of further clinical information the serological findings alone cannot be used to decide whether this was a case of disease or simply contamination.

6.1.3.3.1. Special problems in the interpretation of positive borreliosis serology findings

If specific IgM antibodies to antigens such as those found in the early immune response (OspC, p41) are present in the initial examination, and the investigator is aware of unambiguous clinical findings, the serological finding is compatible with an early stage of Lyme borreliosis. In other circumstances the detection of IgM antibodies alone should be interpreted carefully against the background of the possibility of false positive results. In the absence of additional clinical information, a recent infection (symptomatic or asymptomatic) can only be regarded as confirmed if a subsequent control examination confirms seroconversion (detection of IgG).

In contrast, if the initial examination already shows IgM and IgG antibodies or just IgG antibodies, then from the microbiological viewpoint the serological finding is compatible with a local, disseminated, or persistent *Borrelia* infection (symptomatic or asymptomatic), even in the absence of further information. The decisive factors in the final interpretation of the findings are the nature and number of specific bands in the immunoblot test, and above all the pattern of clinical complaints. In the absence of relevant clinical information it can be concluded that contact with the pathogen has taken place, but it is not possible to say whether manifest disease is present or simply an asymptomatic infection (contamination titers). Detection of specific antibodies of both the IgM and the IgG type does not always correlate with the diagnosis of 'florid Lyme borreliosis'. Depending on the diagnostic method and the *B. burgdorferi* s.l. isolate used for the test, 8-10 % of the average population will give positive antibody titers to *B. burgdorferi* without manifest disease, and the figure will be substantially higher still in high-risk groups with frequent exposure to ticks (up to 50 %; ☞ Section 3.2.1.).

It should also be noted that antibodies (particularly IgG, and less often IgM) can persist for months and sometimes even for years after asymptomatic infections, diseases which resolve spontaneously, and also after antibiotic treatment. On the other hand, rapid treatment in an early stage of the disease can lead to a rapid decline of the antibody titer to below the limit of detection.

It is therefore only possible to draw limited conclusions about the disease stage, or even about the need to treat the infection, on the basis of diagnostic laboratory findings alone. Further clinical information on the disease picture is essential. For all these reasons it is also as a rule not possible to make a definitive assessment of the outcome of treatment on the basis of the results of standard diagnostics.

Apart from the few cases cited above, follow-up serological tests are of little help because neither changes in the titer nor the appearance or disappearance of specific bands in the immunoblot reflect the course of the disease at the time of measurement with sufficient accuracy. Hopefully, new diagnostic systems will in future be able to provide assistance in this respect. So far, however, a detailed medical history and clinical information from the treating doctor are required for this purpose.

6.1.3.4. Detection of specific antibody synthesis in the cerebrospinal fluid in neuroborreliosis

Since specific antibody production can be detected in the cerebrospinal fluid of 60-90 % of patients with *B. burgdorferi* infections of the central nervous system (CNS) or the meninges (☞ Section 5.1.2.2.), depending on the duration of infection and the test system used, in cases of suspected neuroborreliosis the cerebrospinal fluid should be tested for evidence of intrathecal production of *Borrelia* antibodies (☞ Section 6.1.2.). Local IgG synthesis is only associated with corresponding IgM production in about 60 % of the cases. Isolated specific IgM production in the cerebrospinal fluid is rare in neuroborreliosis patients. The test methods of choice are IFA, ELISA, and the immunoblot. In terms of sensitivity and specificity, ELISA and the immunoblot are better than IFT for detecting antibodies in the analysis of the CSF. ELISA in particular allows a substantially more exact quantification of the intrathecal antibody response than titer determination by IFT. On the other hand, ELISA and the immunoblot should be viewed as complementary techniques in CSF diagnostics in terms of their sensitivity and specificity.

CSF-serum antibody index (AI)

The quantity of antibody present in the subarachnoid space depends upon parameters in serum, the permeability of the blood-brain barrier, and the proportion synthesized intrathecally. However, in confirmation of the diagnosis in cases of suspected neuroborreliosis detection of *Borrelia* antibodies in the cerebrospinal fluid alone is not decisive, because the antibodies concerned could have entered the subarachnoid space from the blood due to disturbances in the blood-brain barrier resulting from inflammatory reactions in the meninges. Specific intrathecal synthesis can be demonstrated by the determination of the **CSF-serum antibody index (AI)** in a pair of samples of cerebrospinal fluid and serum obtained on the same day.

> For this purpose the concentrations of the total IgG (IgM, IgA) or of a protein not synthesized in the CSF (e.g. albumin) in serum and cerebrospinal fluid are compared with the concentrations of pathogen-specific antibodies (IgG, IgM, IgA) measured in serum and cerebrospinal fluid.

In practice it is usually sufficient to use the ratio between total-IgG in cerebrospinal fluid and serum as the reference value for the concentration of specific antibodies, and the following formula has been found to be successful for simplified calculation of the AI:

$$\frac{\text{specific Ab - Conc.}[\text{IFA / ELISA}](\text{Liquor}) \times \text{Ig - Conc.}[\text{IgG}](\text{Serum})}{\text{Ig - Conc.}[\text{IgG}](\text{Liquor}) \times \text{specific Ab - Conc.}[\text{IFA / ELISA}](\text{Serum})}$$

The quotient corresponds to the CSF-serum antibody index (AI).

When IFA is used to quantify antibody synthesis on the basis of the CSF-serum antibody index (AI) a quotient of < 2 is regarded as normal. Quotients between 2 and 4 are generally classified as borderline, and quotients greater than 4 are regarded as demonstrating intrathecal production of specific antibodies. However, when an ELISA is used the higher precision of the test systems means that quotients between 1.5 and 2 should be regarded as borderline and quotients > 2 as pathological. The corresponding protein analysis can now be carried out using automatic analyzers, which also permit computer-assisted calculation and evaluation of the findings.

Analysis by immunoblot

The immunoblot technique can be used to diagnose autochthonous antibody production after equalizing the concentrations in cerebrospinal fluid and serum. If, after equalization of the concentrations, the immunoblot test on the cerebrospinal fluid shows significantly stronger specific bands, or bands that are absent from the immunoblot test on the corresponding serum, autochthonous production of *Borrelia* antibodies can be assumed to be occurring in the central nervous system.

Case 5

Meningoradiculitis (stage II)

In the opinion of the neurologists giving treatment, the female patient presented with the classical clinical picture of meningopolyradiculoneuritis (*Bannwarth's disease*). Serological and cerebrospinal fluid tests confirmed the suspected diagnosis. The PCR for *Borrelia* in cerebrospinal fluid and urine, which was also carried out, was negative. As is often the case, the patient did not recall a tick bite. Two weeks of intravenous treatment with ceftriaxone led to a complete cure.

■ Protein analysis

	Serum (mg/dl)	CSF (mg/dl)	Q (CSF/serum) $\times 10^{-3}$	Local synthesis
Alb.	4720	118	25.0	-
IgG	840	30.3	36.1	40 %
IgM	317	12.6	39.7	72 %

6.1. Lyme borreliosis

■ Quotient diagram according to Reiber

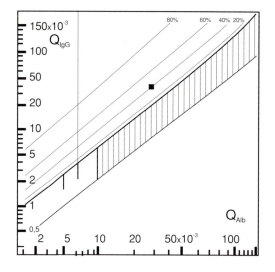

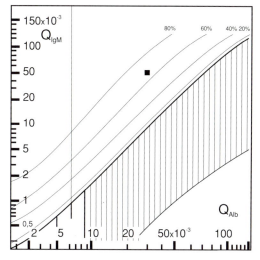

■ Serology

- Serum obtained on August 9, 1997
  - IFA IgG: 1:2560
  - IFA IgM: 1:1280
  - ELISA IgG: 56 U
  - ELISA IgM: +
  - Recombinant immunoblot IgG: p41, p39, p41i
  - Recombinant immunoblot IgM: p100, p41, p39, OspC, p41i
- Cerebrospinal fluid obtained on August 9, 1997
  - IFA IgG: 1:512
  - IFA IgM: 1:16
  - ELISA IgG: 10 U
  - ELISA IgM: +
  - Recombinant immunoblot IgG: p41, p39, p41i
  - Recombinant immunoblot IgM: p41, OspC

■ Antibody index (AI)

- Example of an AI calculation (AI-IgG [ELISA]):

$$AI = \frac{10\ U \times 840\ mg/dl}{30{,}3\ mg/dl \times 56\ U} = \frac{8400}{1696{,}8} = 4{,}9$$

- IgG (IFA): **5.5 positive** (normal value: <2)
- IgM (IFA): 0.3 negative (normal value: <2)
- IgG (ELISA): 4.9 **positive** (normal value: <1.5)

■ Interpretation of the serological findings

IgM and IgG antibodies to *Borrelia*-specific proteins were present in both cerebrospinal fluid and the corresponding serum. The protein analyses in the serum and cerebrospinal fluid revealed a clear disturbance of the blood-brain barrier as an expression of an inflammatory reaction in the meninges ($Q_{alb} \times 10^{-3}$: 25.0 [normal value: < 7]). The signs of an immunological reaction in the CNS were autochthonous immunoglobulin production of 40 % for IgG and 72 % for IgM. The CSF-serum antibody index can be calculated from both IFA and ELISA results by the formula cited above (☞ CSF-serum antibody index). It is noticeable that, in addition to the positive cerebrospinal fluid serology, there was a highly positive CSF-serum antibody index (AI) for IgG, equal to > 5 according to IFA and 4.9 according to ELISA (ENZYGNOST BORRELIOSIS, Dade Behring). In this case the serology confirms infection with *B. burgdorferi* s.l. and involvement of the CNS and its meninges as an expression of an acute organ manifestation of Lyme borreliosis (neuroborreliosis, stage II).

The serological findings in cerebrospinal fluid must always be evaluated in conjunction with the results of cytological and clinicochemical tests (☞ Section 6.1.2.), because on the one hand specific antibodies may be absent in the early phases of neuroborreliosis and, on the other hand, antibody persistence in cerebrospinal fluid over a period of months has been reported even in neuroborreliosis patients who have been given adequate treatment. Specifically, a negative serological finding in the cerebrospinal fluid can only be interpreted as largely excluding borreliosis in the CNS and its meninges if clinical symptoms have already been present for more than 3 months and no signs of acute inflammation are detected in the CSF. In other circumstances the finding should be checked again after about 3-4 weeks. An isolated positive antibody test in cerebrospinal fluid without a corresponding response in serum is detected in about 20 % of cases of neuroborreliosis, depending on the test used and on the calculation procedure.

6.1.3.5. Possible sources of error in serological Lyme borreliosis diagnostics

Despite continuous improvements to the test systems used in borreliosis diagnostics, serological tests continue to give a certain number of false negative and false positive results.

False negative results are particularly common in immunosuppressed patients and in the early stages of Lyme borreliosis, where they result from a delayed antibody response (sensitivity gap). As in the diagnosis of syphilis, false negative findings for specific IgM antibodies occur as a result of negative immunological feedback mechanisms due to high titers of corresponding specific IgG antibodies. Because of the pronounced antigenic heterogeneity it is conceivable that false negative results may sometimes also occur because of the strain causing the infection and the combination of serological tests used, as the antibodies formed may not be recognized by the test (☞ Table 6.12).

False positive reactions caused by cross-reacting antibodies occur both as a result of other bacterial or viral infections and of autoimmune and rheumatic diseases (☞ Table 6.12):

- Cross reactions between various antigens of *Borrelia burgdorferi* s.l. and those of other spirochetes (*T. pallidum* and *T. phagedenis*) and the relapsing fever pathogens *B. hermsii* and *B. duttoni* are known to occur, so pre-absorption of the test sera on Reiter's spirochetes must be carried out, as in syphilis diagnostics, to remove the corresponding nonspecific antibodies. The possibility of existing or prior syphilis can be excluded by screening with the TPHA test. Nonspecific reactions also occur, particularly between certain fairly nonspecific *Borrelia* proteins (p21, flagellin (p41), p66/Oms66, p75) and antibodies to cell-wall constituents of a large number of other gram-negatives (*T. phagedenis, Yersinia enterocolitica 03, Escherichia coli, Campylobacter jejuni, Neisseria meningitidis, Haemophilus influenzae*) and gram-positives (pneumococci, staphylococci) even including tuberculosis bacteria. However, the proteins concerned are mainly fairly nonspecific or nonspecific *Borrelia* proteins. Corresponding nonspecific reactions after prior infections must be taken into consideration when evaluating the diagnostic evidence.

- Nonspecific co-reactions can also occur in borreliosis serology within the context of Epstein-Barr virus or cytomegalovirus infections as a result of polyclonal stimulation of B-cells.

- In addition, false positive reactions are observed in borreliosis serology in the presence of diseases of the rheumatic and autoimmune type and in hematological diseases. Interference by these nonspecific reactions can be largely avoided by pre-absorption on rheumatoid factor absorbent.

Once more it is necessary to draw particular attention to persistent isolated positive IgM findings in the diagnosis of borreliosis. If seroconversion has not occurred at the subsequent control examination it is probable, from the serological viewpoint, that this is a false positive reaction. The reasons for this phenomenon in individual cases often remain unclear.

Information about the antigen products used in the diagnostic tests and appropriate weighting in the evaluation are decisive for a reliable interpretation of serological test results (☞ Table 6.13). However, the use of confirmatory tests of high specificity and sensitivity and careful experimental procedure and evaluation can make differentiation between antibody responses to specific and nonspecific proteins relatively reliable.

6.1.3.6. Need for further standardization of tests

Many serological tests for the detection of Lyme borreliosis are currently on the market, supplied by a large number of manufacturers. The law does not at present require registration of these products. Not unexpectedly, the different methodological approaches themselves result to some extent in substantial quality differences. The use of a technically correct procedure when carrying out the analysis, and the individual operator's experience in the evaluation and assessment of results also play a very pertinent role in the quality of the serological findings, their reproducibility, and their comparability with corresponding findings from other laboratories.

In view of all this, further standardization of the test methods is not just desirable, it is urgently necessary. An important method of regulating the quality of infection serology in general, and of *Borrelia* serology in particular, is regular participation of test laboratories in external quality-control tests with sera which have previously been unambiguously characterized. Each laboratory should also continually validate the diagnostic tests used by running parallel controls and internal laboratory reference sera. Defined antibody panels would be advantageous, particularly to test the proteins separated in the blotting process in respect of their exact location and diagnostic specificity in the whole-cell-antigen immunoblot.

Intensification or loss of specific bands in the immunoblot test, like an increase or decrease in serological titers, can only be regarded as significant if it can be confirmed by appropriate parallel measurements with archived sera. In cases of doubt the doctor requesting the analysis should ask the testing laboratory whether this is done, so that the answer can be taken into account in diagnostic evaluation of the findings. Doubtful or ambiguous cases can usually be clarified by a subsequent examination at a specialist laboratory with experience in the field of borreliosis serology.

The central points of this discussion in essence apply just as much to the other diagnostic procedures used in the borreliosis diagnostics (PCR etc.), though in this case methodological and diagnostic standardization would take even more time.

6.1.3.7. Summary and critical assessment

The many difficulties in standardized implementation and evaluation of diagnostic procedures for **direct pathogen detection** outlined above mean that the widespread use of these methods in routine diagnostics of Lyme borreliosis appears unjustified, especially in view of the doubtful diagnostic value and the high personnel and financial demands. More detailed clinical studies in well characterized groups of patients are still required to determine in particular the diagnostic significance of the PCR. Standardization of the sample collection, sample transport, and the molecular biology techniques is urgently required.

In individual cases the use of the above **special procedures** for **direct pathogen detection** is justified, particularly in difficult differential-diagnostic situations, for example in immunosuppressed patients with inadequate antibody responses or in the very early stages of the disease, as direct detection of the pathogen is of great value in the diagnosis. However, the necessary tests should be carried out in a recognized specialist laboratory.

Consequently, **indirect detection of the pathogen** by detection of specific antibodies with the aid of **standard serological methods** still remains the most important pillar of borreliosis diagnostics in routine microbiological laboratory practice. However, the informative value of the serological findings is strictly limited: in particular, it is not possible to say anything about the need for treatment and certainly not to assess the therapeutic outcome on the basis of diagnostic laboratory findings alone. This requires close cooperation with the doctor giving treatment and the use of additional anamnestic and clinical data.

Above all, it is important to standardize further all procedures used in the diagnosis of Lyme borreliosis to achieve higher quality and comparability of the results.

6.2. Tick-borne encephalitis (TBE)

6.2.1. Principal symptoms and instrumental examinations

TBE must be suspected in the presence of indicative clinical symptoms, especially from the **medical history**, including a sojourn in a known risk area (endemic area) and the double-peak course of the disease with a febrile prodromal phase. Only about 50-60 % of the patients remember a tick bite, so this is of secondary importance.

Although a large proportion of the neurological symptoms are etiologically nonspecific, the ataxia, the other motor disturbances (extrapyramidal symptoms), and especially the distribution of pareses (proximal and in the upper extremities), together with the medical history, can provide valuable evidence about the cause of the disease.

Instrumental investigations are of secondary importance in the diagnosis of TBE. In the absence of focal neurological deficits, only the EEG can provide evidence of an encephalitic course form, and it also has some prognostic value in projecting the course. Electromyography, neurography, transcranial magnetic stimulation, and the evoked potentials can be used for documentation and for prognostic assessment of the course in myelitic and radiculitic forms, but they are of little importance in the primary diagnostics.

Of the available imaging procedures, only the magnetic resonance tomogram should be used. Computed tomography (CT) has not revealed any pathological findings in any of the patients studied so far (n = 110). CT is suitable for exclusion diagnostics in patients with fever-associated cerebral symptoms of unclear etiology. Magnetic resonance tomography yielded pathological findings in 11 % of the cases investigated (n = 78). In the acute stage of the disease the T-2 weighted scan shows signal-rich foci in the thalamus in particular (☞ Fig. 6.8), and less often in the brainstem as well.

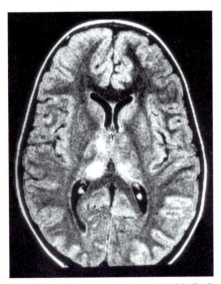

Fig. 6.8: Magnetic resonance tomographic finding in a patient with the encephalitic form of TBE. Typically, signal concentrations are found in the thalamus. (With the kind permission of Dr. Huthwohl, Radiology Department, Offenburg Hospital)

Although detection of these *transient* changes correlates with the severity of the consciousness disturbances it does not correlate with the course form or with the prognosis. In the few cases investigated so far, only patients with clear consciousness disturbances (sopor, coma) show changes of this type, and detection of these changes is very patchy: only a few patients with clear disturbances of consciousness, and not patients who have been comatose for weeks or who have died of the sequelae of the disease, show such changes, even in repeated examinations. On the other hand, many patients with clear signal abnormalities go on to recover completely without residual damage. The recently described relationship between these signal abnormalities and passive immunization is questionable, as the authors concerned did not report any experience relating to these changes in patients who had not been given passive immunization.

6.2.2. Nonspecific laboratory changes in blood and cerebrospinal fluid

Patients in the acute stage of TBE often show pathological inflammation parameters in the serum. Of the patients we have examined:

- 77 % show leukocytosis
  - n = 231
  - median: 12 600/µl
  - range: 9500-31 000/µl
- 87 % show an increased ESR
  - n = 201
  - median: 30 in the first hour (according to Westergren)
  - range: 10-120
- 84 % show increased CRP
  - n = 127
  - median: 3.2 mg/dl
  - range: 0.5-67

Similar observations have been reported in the literature.

Suspected inflammatory disease of the nervous system can be confirmed by an analysis of the cerebrospinal fluid. This typically shows pleocytosis, at first mainly granulocytic but later mainly lymphocytic. Mild to moderate disturbance of the blood-brain barrier is observed in 70-80 % of the cases. Table 6.14 shows a collection of typical pathological findings in the cerebrospinal fluid of patients with TBE.

6.2.3. Microbiological diagnostics

- After Lyme borreliosis, spring-summer encephalitis TBE, caused by a virus of the same name, a member of the family Flaviviridae (☞ Section 2.2.), with its two regional subtypes:
- subtype 1 (which causes CEE) and
- subtype 2 (which causes RTBE),

is the most important disease transmitted by ticks of the genus Ixodes in Europe. The methods available for microbiological diagnosis of the pathogen are direct detection, e.g. by electron microscopy or isolation of the virus, and indirect confirmation of infection by serological detection of specific antibodies (☞ Table 6.15).

Direct detection techniques (virus detection)	Indirect detection techniques (antibody detection)
• RT-PCR • Electron microscopy • Virus culture	• ELISA • Immunoblot • Hemagglutination inhibition test (HIT) • Virus neutralization test (NT) • Complement-fixation reaction (CFR)

Table 6.15: Direct and indirect test methods in microbiological TBE diagnostics. The standard test method for diagnosing TBE in routine microbiological laboratories is **ELISA** for the detection of specific antibodies. The other methods are more difficult and are only indicated in special cases

Classical procedures such as culture of the virus, electron microscopy, the hemagglutination inhibition test (HIT), the virus neutralization test (NT), and the CFR have fallen increasingly into the background in view the advances in the ELISA technique. For a few years now it has also been possible to detect the virus directly by the reverse-transcriptase polymerase chain reaction (RT-PCR).

6.2.3.1. Direct microbiological methods (detection of the virus)

6.2.3.1.1. Culture of the virus and electron microscopy

Samples of blood and cerebrospinal fluid collected under sterile conditions during the early viremic phase of the disease are suitable for viral cultures and for examination by electron microscopy. Blood should be heparinized after collection. Viruses can be cultured from clinical material for example in chick embryo cell cultures. Although multiplication of the virus does not cause a cytopathic effect in this system, a positive culture can be recognized by the increased secretion of interferon or by direct IFA. Blood or cerebrospinal fluid can be used directly for the culture after a check for sterility, but biopsy material should first be equilibrated with 10 % inactivated normal human serum free from TBE antibodies. Specimen material which is not processed at once must be deep-frozen at -70°C. Only specialist laboratories carry out direct virus detection. The technique is only of importance for reliable confirmation of infection in early stages of the disease and in unclear neurological pictures where TBE is suspected and the serology is negative. Attempts at direct detec-

Parameter	Normal value	Pathological finding in	Median	Range
Pleocytosis (cells/µl)	< 5	100 %[1]	85	6-1000
Total protein (mg/l)	< 450	80 %[1]	650	250-2200
Albumin quotient ($\times 10^{-3}$)	< 8	70 %[2]	10	3-40
IgM synthesis (%)	0	50 %[2]	30	5-90
IgG synthesis (%)	0	25 %[2]	15	5-60
IgA synthesis (%)	0	12 %[2]	15	5-70

[1] Evaluation of 500 cerebrospinal fluid tests. [2] Evaluation of 100 cerebrospinal fluid tests

Table 6.14: Incidence of pathological findings in the cerebrospinal fluid in TBE

tion are also indicated in TBE infections following excessively acute courses.

Both culture techniques and the examination of clinical material (brain biopsy) by electron microscopy are indicated in post-mortem diagnostics for definitive establishment of TBE in fatal infections.

After successful culture it is possible for specialist laboratories to use NT, HIT, or IFT to identify the subtype. Distinguishing between the CEE virus and the RTBE virus also requires oligopeptide analyses on the viral proteins.

6.2.3.1.2. Direct detection of TBE virus by RT-PCR

The advances in modern molecular biology mean that pathogens can be diagnosed directly in clinical material by detecting their genetic material with the aid of the PCR and nested-PCR. In the case of DNA viruses, detection of the viral genetic material is carried out using the molecular-biology methods already described in detail in an earlier section (☞ Section 6.1.3.1.4.). However, the genome of the TBE virus, like that of all flaviviruses, is organized in the form of a single stranded RNA (☞ Section 2.2.2.). A modification of the PCR method therefore initially makes use of a special viral enzyme, the so-called reverse transcriptase (RT). This enzyme, an RNA-dependent DNA-polymerase, together with a special primer, is able to transcribe the single-stranded RNA matrix of the viral genome to give the complementary single strand of DNA (c-DNA). This reaction is followed by cyclic synthesis of new DNA in a manner analogous to conventional PCR (☞ Section 6.1.3.1.4.). This procedure is known as RT-PCR and is used in virological diagnostics for direct detection of RNA viruses.

Direct detection of the TBE virus in blood (citrated or edetated blood), cerebrospinal fluid, or biopsy specimens during the viremic phase by this very sensitive and specific molecular-biology method is so far used only occasionally and by specialist laboratories.

6.2.3.2. Indirect detection methods (detection of antibodies)

NT, HIT, CFR, and TBE-specific ELISAs and immunoblots can be used for the assessment of the immunological status and the serological detection of antibodies where there is a clinical suspicion of a recent TBE infection. Although the first two of these serological tests can be used to detect TBE antibodies, they are technically difficult and are not good enough for class-specific immunglobulin analysis, particularly for the specific detection of IgM. As a result, the differential assessment of the duration of infection cannot be carried out, or can only be carried out on the basis of follow-up examinations. HIT and CFR no longer play any role in serodiagnostics in the routine microbiological laboratories. NT is methodologically demanding, and is only used in specialist laboratories to resolve special questions (differentiation of cross-reactions after infection or inoculation against other flaviviruses, identification and typing of virus isolates).

Because of its good practicality and its sensitivity and specificity, **ELISA** is currently the method of choice in the early and rapid serological diagnostics of TBE in serum and cerebrospinal fluid. The **immunoblot** (☞ Section 6.1.3.2.2.), another very sensitive and specific test for detecting TBE antibodies, is used in specialist laboratories, but is technically more difficult than the ELISA and so far only of subordinate importance in TBE diagnostics.

6.2.3.2.1. ELISA

The ELISA technique (☞ Section 6.1.3.2.2.) offers a very sensitive and specific method for detecting IgM and IgG antibodies in the diagnosis of TBE while requiring relatively little work. New techniques also seek to provide better information about the time of infection by measuring the strength of the antigen-antibody binding (avidity) in the ELISA after denaturation with chaotropic reagents (e.g. urea). Antibodies of low avidity and weak antigen binding correspond to an early phase of infection. By contrast, high-avidity antibodies with strong antigen-binding are only formed in the later stages of the disease or after prior infections, and are associated with immunity to the pathogen.

For detection of IgG, depending on the test manufacturer, it may be possible to convert the result into test-specific units. Specific IgM antibodies can be detected by so-called 'indirect' ELISA, after neutralization of possibly interfering IgG antibodies (e.g. by rheumatoid factor absorption), or by the 'immunometric' ELISA method. The IgG-ELISA results correlate well with the virus-neutralizing antibody titers in NT in checks of the success of inoculation. In the presence of virus-specific antibodies, by using this method it is possible both to obtain reliable information about the immunological status and to give an opinion about the possibility of a recent infection with adequate specificity and sensitivity from a single blood sample. Cross-reactions after infection or inoculation with other flaviviruses do, however, occur, and may need to be excluded.

6.2.3.2.2. Antibody kinetics and interpretation of findings in the course of an TBE infection

The antibody formation and the course of the immune response after an infection with the TBE virus corresponds to those after other viral infections. The main immunogen for the formation of protective antibodies is coat protein E from the surface of the virus (☞ Section 2.2.3.).

It is possible to detect specific IgM antibodies suggesting a recent infection about 7-10 days after the infection of individuals having a normal immunity status. The formation of IgG antibodies follows from the second week. Proof of a recent infection is provided by the simultaneous detection of specific IgM and IgG antibodies or a 4-fold increase in the specific IgG titer in serum. The absence of an IgM response or a persistence of IgM antibodies is seldom reported. After post-exposure passive immunization the formation of antibodies can be delayed, so a control serology may be indicated after 10 to 14 days if the finding is unclear. While the IgM antibodies and complement-activating antibodies mostly disappear over a period of weeks or months, the IgG persist for life after a wild infection (permanent immunity) and can be diagnosed with the aid of serological test systems. Isolated IgG antibodies are an expression of a former infection or inoculation. In the endemic regions of Europe TBE antibodies are found in about 14-42 % of the population. This correlates with the prevalence of TBE infection in the tick population in the endemic region. The normal kinetics of the antibody response after TBE infection are illustrated in Fig. 6.9.

A class-specific immunglobulin analysis of the immune response is essential for a reliable assessment of the state of immunity and indirect detection of a recent infection. Interpretation problems occur after active TBE inoculation, since IgM can sometimes be detected for a fairly long time in such cases. Because of the antigenic similarity to other flaviviruses, cross reactions may occur after yellow-fever inoculation or due to infections with other *Flaviviridae*. This possibility should be excluded on the basis of the medical history.

In clinically unclear neurological disease pictures the medical laboratory should also consider the possibility of rare cases of a concomitant *Borrelia* infection.

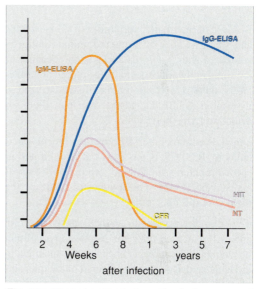

Fig. 6.9: Normal antibody formation in the course of an TBE infection (modified according to Blessing, 1996)

6.2.3.2.3. Detection of antibodies in the cerebrospinal fluid in TBE

Like Lyme borreliosis, TBE infection of the CNS produces a typical pattern of findings in tests on the cerebrospinal fluid. The decisive factor in serological detection of an TBE infection in the CNS is the detection of specific IgG and/or IgM antibodies. As in other infectious diseases of the CNS (e.g. neuroborreliosis), the CSF-serum antibody index (AI) can be used for this purpose (☞ Section 6.1.3.4.). When an ELISA is used to detect antibodies, an AI of 1.5 to 2 counts as borderline, and an AI > 2 as pathological. Once again, when evaluating the serological findings it is important to know the other microbiological, chemical laboratory, and cytological test results (☞ Section 6.2.2.), because specific antibodies may be absent in the early stages of the disease.

6.2.3.3. Critical assessment

The standard TBE diagnostics in routine microbiological laboratory practice are now largely based on serological detection of specific antibodies (IgM, IgG) by the ELISA technique (indirect detection of infection). In the majority of cases both the immunological status (successful inoculation) and the duration of infection (recent or older infection) can be determined with sufficiently good reliability.

Because of the smaller variability of virus isolates and small number of immunodominant antigens compared with *B. burgdorferi* s.l., and because of the small number of vaccine and antigen manufacturers, there is a greater degree of standardization in serological TBE diagnostics than in methods for detecting Lyme borreliosis.

Direct detection of the TBE virus in clinical specimens by RT-PCR is possible, but it is limited to special problems and is so far offered only by specialist laboratories. The diagnostic value of the method is still uncertain.

The other direct and indirect methods of detection and differentiation (electron microscopy, culture, immunoblot) are mostly expensive and technically difficult, so they are only indicated in the microbiological TBE diagnostics in exceptional cases.

References

Amberger W., Rumpl E. (1994). Klinisch-elektroenzephalographische Korrelationen bei der Frühsommer-Meningoenzephalitis. EEG-EMG 25: 190-195

Bayer M.E., Zhang L., Bayer M.H. (1996). *Borrelia burgdorferi* DNA in the urine of treated patients with chronic Lyme-disease symptoms. A PCR study of 97 cases. Infection 24: 347-353

Blessing J. (1996). Frühsommer-Menigoenzephalitis (FSME)-Virus. In: Virusdiagnostik, Horstmann T. (Hrsg.), Blackwell Wissenschaftsverlag, Berlin: 188-200

Blumenthal W., Ackermann R., Schottky A. (1970). Zentraleuropäische Enzephalitis unter dem Bild einer lumbalen Poliomyelitis. Med. Klinik 65: 153-156

Bodemann H., Hoppe-Seyler P., Blum H., Herkel L. (1980). Schwere und ungünstige Verlaufsformen der Zeckenenzephalitis (FSME) 1979 in Freiburg. Dtsch. Med. Wschr. 105: 921-924

Bodemann H., Pausch J., Schmitz H., Hoppe-Seyler P. (1977). Die Zeckenenzephalitis (FSME) als Labor-Infektion. Med.Welt 28: 1779-1781

Brade V., Albert S. (1997). Mikrobiologische Diagnostik bei Lyme-Borreliose. In: Prange H., Bitsch A. (Hrsg.): Bakterielle ZNS-Erkrankungen bei systemischen Infektionen. Steinkopf-Verlag, Darmstadt: 99-109

Brede H.D. (1997). FSME - Ein Situationsbericht. Notabene Medici 4: 165-167

Bundesgesundheitsinstitut für gesundheitlichen Verbraucherschutz und Veterinärmedizin (BgVV) und Robert Koch Institut (RKI). (1997). Frühsommer-Meningoenzephalitis (FSME) - Erkennung und Verhütung - Merkblatt für Ärzte. Der Mikrobiologe 7: 16-18

CDC. (1995). Recommendations for test performance and interpretation from the second national conference on serologic diagnosis of Lymedisease. JAMA 274: 937

Chary-Valckenaere I., Jaulhac B., Monteil H., Pourel J. (1997). Diagnosis of Lymedisease. current difficulties and prospects. Rev. Rheum. [Engl. Ed.] 62: 271-280

Curtin S.M., Pennington T.H. (1995). The diagnosis of Lyme-disease. J. R. Soc. Med. 88: 248-250

Figueroa R., Bracero L.A., Aguero-Rosenfeld M., Beneck D., Coleman J., Schwartz I. (1996). Confirmation of *Borrelia burgdorferi* spirochetes by PCR in placentas of women with reactive serology for Lyme Antibodies. Gynecol. Obste. Invest. 41: 240-243

Flisiak R., Kalinowska A., Bobrowska E., Prokopowicz D. (1996). Enzyme immunoassay in the diagnosis of Lyme borreliosis. Rocz. Akad. Med. Bialymst. 41: 83-89

Fulop L., Barrett A.D.T., Phillpotts R., Martin K., Leslie D., Titball R.W. (1993). Rapid identification of flaviviruses based on NS5 gene sequences. J. Virol. Meth. 44: 179-188

Gassmann C., Bauer G. (1997). Avidity determination of IgG directed against tick-borne encephalitis virus improves detection of current infections. J. Med. Virol. 51: 242-251

Gresikova M., Kaluzuva M. (1997). Biology of tick-borne encephalitis virus. Act. Virol. 41: 115-124

Grinschgl G. (1955). Virus meningo-encephalitis in Austria. Clinical features, pathology and diagnosis. Bull. Wld. Hlth. Org. 12: 535-564

Gunther G., Haglund M., Lindquist L., Forsgren M., Skoldenberg B. (1997). Tick-bone encephalitis in Sweden in relation to aseptic meningo-encephalitis of other etiology: a prospective study of clinical course and outcome. J. Neurol. 244: 230-238

Hamann-Brand A., Breitner S., Schulze J., Brade V. (1995). Laboratory diagnosis of Lyme disease. Biotest Bulletin 5: 127-142

Hamann-Brand A., Flondor M., Brade V. (1994). Evaluation of a passive Hemaglutination assay as screening test and of a recombinant immunoblot as confirmatory test for serological diagnosis of Lyme-disease. Eur. J. Clin. Microbiol. Infect. Dis. 13: 572-575

Hauser U., Krahl H., Peters H., Fingerle V., Wilske B. (1998). Impact of strain heterogeneity on Lyme disease serology in Europe: Comparison of enzyme-linked immunosorbent assays using different species of *Borrelia burgdorferi* sensu lato. J. Clin. Micobiol. 36: 427-436

Hauser U., Lehnert G., Lobentanzer R., Wilske B. (1997). Interpretation criteria for standardized western blots for three European species of *Borrelia burgdorferi* sensu lato. J. Clin. Microbiol. 35: 1433-1444

Holzmann H., Kundi M., Stiasny K., Kunz C., Heinz F.X. (1995). Korrelation und Bewertung von Antikörpernachweissystemen zur Kontrolle des FSME-Impferfolges. In: Durch Zecken übertragene Erkrankungen: FSME und Lyme-Borreliose. Süss J. (Hrsg.). Weller-Verlag: 44-47

Hornig C.R., Busse O., Dorndorf W. (1984). Charakteristic cerebrospinal fluid findings and clinical aspects of lymphocytic meningoradiculitis. Klin. Wochenschr. 62: 30-34

Hunfeld KP., Allwinn R., Albert S., Brade V., Doerr HW. (1998). Serologically proven double infection with tick-borne encephalitis virus (TBEV) and *Borrelia burgdorferi*. J. Lab. Med. 22: 409-413

Issakainen J., Gnehm H.E., Lucchini G.M., Zbinden R. (1996). Value of clinical symptoms, intrathecal specific antibody production and PCR in CSF in the diagnosis of childhood Lyme neuroboreliosis. Klin. Pediatr. 208: 106-109

Kaiser R., Holzmann H., Heinz F.X. (1998). Tick-borne encephalitis: Relevance of laboratory data for prognosis. in preparation

Kaiser R., Kern A., Fressle R., Steinbrecher A., Omran H., Malzacher V., Kügler D., Kampa D., Batsford S. (1996). Zeckenvermittelte Erkrankungen in Baden-Würtemberg. Epidemiologische Studie zur Häufigkeit stationär behandlungsbedürftiger FSME- und Borreliose-Erkrankungen im Jahr 1995. Münch. Med. Wschr. 138: 647-652

Kamradt T., Krause A., Priem S., Burmester G.R. (1998). Die Lyme-Arthritis: Klinik, Diagnose und Therapie. Dt. Ärztebl. 95: A-214-219

Kießig S.T., Abel U., Heinz F.X., Enzensberger O., Risse P., Friedrich J. (1996). Methodenvergleich für die Diagnostik der FSME unter Einbeziehung des Western-Blots und anderer Referenzmethoden im Hinblick auf die Festlegung von Schwellenwerten. In: Durch Zecken übertragene Erkrankungen: FSME und Lyme-Borreliose. Süss J. (Hrsg.), Weller-Verlag Schrießheim: 48-66

Kießig S.T., Abel U., Risse P., Friedrich J., Heinz F.X., Kunz C.H. (1993). Bestimmung von Schwellenwerten (cut of) bei Enzymimmunoassys am Beispiel des FSME-ELISA. Klin. Lab. 11: 877-886

Kristoferitsch W., Stanek G., Kunz C. (1986). Doppelinfektion mit Frühsommermeningoenzephalitis (FSME)- Virus und *Borrelia burgdorferi*. Dtsch. Med. Wschr. 111: 861-864

Kruger H., Heim E., Schuknecht B., Scholz S. (1991). Acute and chronic neuroborreliosis with and without CNS involvement: a clinical, MRI, and HLA study of 27 cases. J. Neurol. 238: 271-280

Ledue T.B., Collins M., Craig W.Y. (1996). New laboratory guidelines for serologic diagnosis of Lyme-disease: evaluation of the two-test protocol. J. Clin. Microbiol. 34: 2343-2350

Liedke W., Opalka B., Zimmermann C.W., Schmid E. (1994). Different methods of sample preparation influence sensitivity of *Mycobacterium tuberculosis* and *Borrelia burgdorferi* PCR. PCR Methods Applic. 3: 301-304

Lorenzl S., Pfister H.W., Padovan C., Yousry T. (1996). MRI abnormalities in tick-borne encephalitis. Lancet 347: 698-699

Magnarelli L.A. (1995). Current status of laboratory diagnosis for Lyme disease. Am. J. Med. 98 (Suppl. 4A): 10-12

Magnarelli L.A., Fikrig E., Padula S.J., Anderson J.F., Flavell R.A. (1996). Use of recombinant antigens of *Borrelia burgdorferi* in serologic tests for diagnosis of Lyme borreliosis. J. Clin. Microbiol. 34: 237-240

Masuzawa T., Komikado T., Yanagihra Y. (1997). RCR-restriction fragment length polymorphism analysis of the ospC gene for detection of mixed culture and fore epidemiological typing of *Borrelia burgdorferi* sensu stricto. Clin. Diagn. Lab. Immunol. 4: 60-63

Mosuni M.S., Kaiser R., Motamedi S., Spöttl F. (1974). Frühsommer-Meningoenzephalitis im Bezirk Schärding in den Jahren 1972 und 1973. Wiener Klinische Wochenschrift 86: 593-596

Mouritsen C.L., Wittwer C.T., Litwin C.M., Yang L., Weis J.L., Martins T.B., Jaskowski T.D., Hill H.R. (1996). Polymerase chain reaktion detection of Lyme disease: Correlation with clinical manifestations and serological responses. Am. J. Clin. Pathol. 105: 647-654

Norman G.L., Antig J.F., Bigaignon G., Hogrefe W.R. (1996). Serodiagnosis of Lyme borreliosis by *Borrelia burgdorferi* sensu stricto, *B. garinii* and *B. afzelii* western blots (immunoblots). J. Clin. Microbiol. 34: 1732-1738

Oschmann P. (1989). Diagnose, Therapie und Verlauf der akuten und chronischen Borreliose. Inaugural Dissertation an der Bayerischen Julius-Maximilian-Universität

Oschmann P., Dorndorf W., Hornig C., Schäfer C., Wellensiek H.J., Pflughaupt K.W. (1998). Stages and syndromes of neuroborreliosis. J. Neurol. 245: 262-272

Oschmann P., Wellensiek H.J., Dorndorf W., Pflughaupt K.W. (1997). Intrathecal synthesis of specific antibodies in neuroborreliosis: Comparison of immunoblotting, indirect immunofluorescence assay and enzyme-linked immunosorbent assay. J. Lab. Med. 21: 528-534

Oschmann P., Wellensiek H.J., Zhong W., Dorndorf W., Pflughaupt K.W. (1997). Relationship between the *Borrelia burgdorferi* specific immune response and different stages and syndromes in neuroborreliosis. Infection 25: 292-297

Preac-Mursic V. (1992). In vitro und in vivo Antibiotikaempfindlichkeit von *Borrelia burgdorferi*: Therapeutische Folgerungen. In: Lyme-Borreliose. Hassler D. (Hrsg.). Medizin Verlag München: 133-143

Priem S., Rittig M.G., Kamradt T., Burmester G.R., Krause A. (1997). An optimized PCR leads to rapid and high detection of *Borrelia burgdorferi* in patients with Lyme borreliosis. J. Clin. Microbiol. 35: 685-690

Schmidt B.L. (1997). PCR in diagnosis of human *Borrelia burgdorferi* infections. Clin. Microbiol. Rev. 10: 185-201

Schwan T.G., Schrumpf M.E., Hinnebusch B.J., Anderson D.E., Konkel M.E. (1996). GIpQ: an antigen for serological dicrimination between relapsing fever and Lyme borreliosis. J. Clin. Microbiol. 34: 2483-2492

Selzer E.G., Shapiro E.D. (1996). Misdiagnosis of Lyme disease: When not to order serologic tests. Pediatr. Infect. Dis. J. 15: 762-763

Skare J.T., Mirzabekov T.A., Shang E.S., Blanko D.R., Erdjument-Bromage H., Bunikis J., Bergström S., Tempst P., Kagan B.L., Miller J.N., Lovett M.A. (1997). The Oms66 (p66) protein is a *Borrelia burgdorferi* porin. Infect. Immun. 65: 3654-3661

Stanek G., O'Connell S., Cimmino M., Aberer E., Kristoferitsch W., Granström M., Guy E., Gray J. (1996). European Union concerted action on risk assessment in Lyme borreliosis: clinical case definitions for Lyme borreliosis. Wien. Klin. Wochenschr. 108 (23): 741-747

Steere A.C. (1997). Diagnosis and treatment of Lyme arthritis. Med. Clin. North. Am. 81: 179-194

Svenungsson B., Lindh G. (1997). Lyme borreliosis - an overdiagnosed disease? Infection 25: 140-143

Tomazic J., Poljac M., Popovic P., Maticic M., Beovic B., Ausic-Zupanc T., Lotric S., Jereb M., Pikelj F., Gale N. (1997). Tick-borne-encephalitis: Possibly a fatal disease in its acute stage. PCR amplification of TBE-RNA from post mortem brain tissue. Infection 25: 41-43

Tumani H., Nolken G., Reiber H. (1995). Relevance of cerebrospinal fluid variables for early diagnosis of neuroborreliosis. J. Neurol. 37: 749-753

Valdueza J., Weber J., Harms L., Bock A. (1997). Severe tick borne encephalomyelits after tick bite and passive immunisation. JNNP 345: 593-594

Valsangicomo C., Balmelli T., Piffaretti J.C. (1996). A nested polymerase chain reaction for the detection of *Borrelia burgdorferi* sensu lato based on a multiple sequence analysis of the hbb gene. FEMS Microbiol. Letters 136: 25-29

Verdon M.E., Sigal L. (1997). Recognition and management of Lyme disease. Am. Fam. Phys. 56: 427-436

Wilske B., Fingerle V., Herzer P., Hofmann A., Lehnert G., Peters H., Pfister H.W., Preac-Mursic V., Weber K. (1993). Recombinant immunoblot in the serodiagnosis of Lyme borreliosis: Comparison with indirect immunofluorescence and enzyme-linked immunosorbent assay. Med. Microbiol. Immunol. 182: 255-270

Wilske B., Fingerle V., Preac-Mursic V., Jauris-Heipke S., Hofmann A., Loy H., Pfister H.W., Rössler D., Soutschek E. (1994). Immunoblot using rekombinant antigens derived from different genospecies of *Borrelia burgdorferi* sensu lato. Med. Microbiol. Immunol. 183: 43-59

Wilske B., Preac-Mursic V. (1993). Microbiological diagnosis of Lyme borreliosis. In: Aspects of Lyme borreliosis. Weber K., Burgdorfer W. (Eds.). Springer Verlag, Berlin: 257-299

Zhong W., Oschmann P., Wellensiek H.J. (1997). Detection and preliminary characterization of circulating immune complexes in patients with Lyme disease. Med. Microbiol. Immunol. (Berl) 1986: 153-158

Therapy and prognosis

7. Therapy and prognosis

7.1. Lyme borreliosis

Decades before the discovery of *B. burgdorferi* as the pathogen that causes Lyme borreliosis, various manifestations of this disease such as

- erythema chronicum migrans (*Hellström*, 1951)
- acrodermatitis chronica atrophicans (Svartz, 1946), and
- meningopolyneuritis (*Hellström*, 1951)

were already being treated successfully with penicillin. However, clinical studies have since demonstrated not only a frequent occurrence of relapses, late complications, and delayed cures despite adequate penicillin therapy, but also the superiority of other antibiotics over penicillin.

> Despite the many studies that have been carried out recently, there is still no standard treatment for Lyme borreliosis and further improvements are necessary.

Current therapeutic strategies are largely founded on in-vitro studies with pathogen isolates, on insights gained from animal models, and on clinical experience.

7.1.1. Therapy

7.1.1.1. Therapeutic principles

In all stages of Lyme borreliosis *B. burgdorferi* can be detected microscopically, by culture, or by PCR. The factors that must be taken into consideration in treating the disease are the intrinsic sensitivity of the pathogen, the tissue penetration of the antibiotic, and pathogen-specific characteristics such as a long generation time (7-20 h in vitro) and the development of "persister" forms (☞ Table 7.1). What is also important is a sufficiently long course of antibiotic at a sufficiently high dosage.

> - Long generation time of the pathogen (7-20 h)
> - Intracellular localization of the pathogen
> - Development of "persister" forms
> - Residence of the pathogen in tissues with a poor blood supply (e.g. synovia)
> - Blood-CSF (blood-brain) barrier
> - Tissue penetration of the antibiotic
> - Varying antibiotic resistance of different pathogen strains

Table 7.1: Factors important in choosing the type, dose, and duration of antibiotic treatment

In vitro the most effective antibiotics are the macrolides (azithromycin, roxithromycin, erythromycin) and third-generation cephalosporins (cefotaxime, ceftriaxone; ☞ Table 7.2 and Section 6.1.3.1.3.). Far behind these come doxycycline and amoxicillin, with penicillins exhibiting high minimal inhibitory concentrations. *Borreliae* are primarily resistant to aminoglycosides, trimethoprim/sulfamethoxazole, and gyrase inhibitors. In experimental animal studies the activity of erythromycin was comparable with that of penicillin G, with poor inhibition of the pathogen. The newer macrolides (e.g. roxithromycin) seem superior here, although clinical experience is very limited. For most antibiotics, if the meninges are not inflamed, low penetration of the cerebrospinal fluid is the limiting factor. The third-generation cephalosporins are advantageous in such cases. Of the other antibiotics, only with

Antibiotic	Dose	Concentration in CSF [µg/ml]		Minimal inhibitory concentration (range for various isolates)
		inflamed	not inflamed	
Penicillin G	5×10^6 IU, i.v.	0.9	0.15	0.5-8.0
	10×10^6 IU, i.v.	4.8	0.8	
Amoxicillin	1 g, i.v.	3.0	0.3	0.5-1.9
Ceftriaxone	2 g, i.v.	5.4	0.43	0.03-0.6
Cefotaxime	2 g, i.v.	15.2	0.3	0.06-0.10

Table 7.2: Minimal inhibitory concentrations of various antibiotics and their CSF penetration

doxycycline can borderline therapeutic concentrations be expected. The development of vasculitic changes can also hinder tissue penetration. Moreover, treatment of borreliosis is complicated by certain characteristics of the pathogen. *B. burgdorferi* divides very slowly, and under unfavorable conditions the division times observed in vitro could conceivably be distinctly exceeded in vivo, necessitating long treatment times with uniform and sufficiently high antibiotic levels, as β-lactam antibiotics are active only during the division phase. Furthermore, in *Borrelia* infections the action of antibiotics can lead to the development of persisters, viable bacteria that have survived lethal doses but are still sensitive at the end of the antibiotic treatment. What has not been adequately investigated is how often the persister forms are responsible for the occurrence of relapses and delayed cures. An important practical consideration is the observation of distinct differences in antibiotic sensitivity both between *Borrelia garinii* and *Borrelia afzelii* and between different strains of the same species, which may be the reason for observed treatment failures. Antibiotic sensitivity tests are not helpful, as it is rarely possible to isolate the causative agent.

7.1.1.2. Pragmatic therapy

A generally accepted antibiotic treatment regimen has yet to gain common currency, and all treatment recommendations are essentially provisional. The proposals listed below (☞ Table 7.3) are based on original publications and on our own experience. To avoid giving inappropriate treatment, stage- and syndrome-oriented therapy is advisable.

7.1.1.2.1. Therapy of stage I

In most cases this means erythema migrans or, in rare cases, lymphadenosis cutis benigna. Oral therapy is generally sufficient if the patient can be relied upon to take the drug as instructed. Suitable regimens are

- doxycycline (2 × 100 mg oral),
- amoxicillin (3 × 1000 mg oral), or
- cefuroxime (2 × 500 mg oral),

in each case for 2-3 weeks. With regard to the very good in-vitro activity of macrolide antibiotics,

Stage	Manifestation	Antibiotic	Dose/day	Route	Duration	Experience
I	Erythema migrans	doxycycline[1]	2 × 100 mg	p.o.	14 days	broad
	Lymphadenosis cutis benigna	amoxicillin	3 × 1000 mg (children: 3 × 10 mg/kg)	p.o.	14 days	broad
		cefuroxime	2 × 500 mg	p.o.	14 days	little
		roxithromycin	3 × 500 mg	p.o.	14 days	little
		azithromycin	2 × 500 mg	p.o.	5 days	very little
II	Neuroborreliosis, Lyme arthritis[2], Lyme carditis[2], ophthalmo-borreliosis[2]	cefotaxime	3 × 2 g (children: 3 × 30 mg/kg)	i.v.	14 days	broad
		ceftriaxone	1 × 2 g (children: 60 mg/kg)	i.v.	14 days	broad
		doxycycline[1]	2 × 100 mg	i.v./p.o.	14 days	little
III	Neuroborreliosis, acrodermatitis chronica atrophicans[2]	cefotaxime	3 × 2 g	i.v.	21 days	broad
			2 × (3 × 4 g; pulse therapy)[3]	i.v.	6-8 cycles	little
		ceftriaxone	1 × 2 g	i.v.	21 days	broad
		doxycycline	2 × 100 mg	i.v./p.o.	21 days	little

[1]in patients allergic to β-lactam antibiotics, contraindicated in children under 9 years; [2]oral treatment with doxycycline or cefuroxime can be tried in uncomplicated cases; [3]see Table 7.8

Table 7.3: Stage- and manifestation-adapted therapy of Lyme borreliosis

there is experience e.g. with azithromycin (2×0.5 g oral). Even despite therapy, treatment failure can occur in around 1-3 % of the cases, with the development of neurological and rheumatological symptoms. Patients in whom corresponding symptoms (e.g. headaches, fever, arthralgias) pointing to a generalization of the infection were already present prior to treatment are particularly predisposed. In such cases the bacterium may have already colonized the subarachnoid space or the joints, where oral antibiotics achieve only borderline therapeutic concentrations. An alternative to frequent clinical monitoring in these patients is intravenous treatment with a third-generation cephalosporin. Usually, good regression of the cutaneous efflorescences is achieved within days of commencing treatment. In the absence of treatment the course of the condition is longer and the incidence of late complications higher, at around 8 % (Europe). The longer the latency period after the development of EM, the less likely the progression to stages II and III. It therefore seems justifiable to suspend treatment provisionally if no new symptoms have developed during the 6-month period following disappearance of the EM. Monitoring of the clinical course and counseling of the patient is, however, recommended. Disappearance of the EM even without treatment is no proof that the infection has gone, and the indication for treatment continues to apply in principle.

7.1.1.2.2. Therapy of stage II

Rheumatological, cardiac, ophthalmological, and neurological clinical pictures can all occur in stage II. On the basis of pathophysiological considerations, poor penetration of the cerebrospinal fluid, and the low absorption of oral antibiotics, preference is generally given to intravenous antibiotic therapy.

Systematic studies have been carried out mainly in patients with neuroborreliosis. Debate on the benefit of antibiotic treatment was sparked by a Würzburg research group, which conducted a retrospective study of 57 untreated patients and 66 patients who had been given antibiotics (penicillin G, in some cases doxycycline), covering posttreatment periods ranging from 5 to 27 years. The authors found no difference either between the frequencies of the mostly slight residual symptoms (dysesthesias, pareses) in the two groups (around 40 %) or between the times taken for the cerebrospinal fluid to become normal. None of the 113 patients went on to develop the chronic form of the condition. In smaller prospective studies (22-75 patients) no clear differences were discernible between penicillin G, doxycycline, ceftriaxone, and cefotaxime. Treatment failures have been reported for all antibiotics. These findings can be explained by the relatively good prognosis in neuroborreliosis, with a statistically detectable effect on the spontaneous course to be expected only in larger groups of patients. For some of the *Borrelia* strains isolated it must be assumed that penicillin therapy will be ineffective (☞ Table 7.2), and the use of third-generation cephalosporins (e.g. cefotaxime 3×2 g/day) seems advisable. Patients known to be allergic to β-lactams can be given intravenous doxycycline (2×100 mg daily). Experience with macrolide antibiotics in stage II is limited. Except for cases of Lyme arthritis there have not been any studies of other organ manifestations of stage II. Here also treatment with a third-generation cephalosporin seems advisable. In uncomplicated cases of Lyme arthritis or ophthalmoborreliosis some authors have recommended trying an oral antibiotic (e.g. doxycycline) first, reserving intravenous antibiotic treatment for cases that prove to be refractory.

Administration of steroids prior to antibiotic therapy can promote the development of chronic arthritis which is difficult to treat, and should therefore be avoided in all cases. Nonsteroidal anti-inflammatories present no problems as concomitant medication.

In rare cases of treatment failure patients with chronic arthritis may benefit from synovectomy.

7.1.1.2.3. Therapy of stage III

Even in the third stage of Lyme borreliosis the clinical course can still respond to antibiotics. What has yet to be clarified is the role of secondary immunological mechanisms. In tertiary neuroborreliosis immunosuppressants have been used both alone and in combination with intravenous and intrathecal antibiotics. Immunosuppressants on their own were not effective on a long-term basis, a lasting effect on the disease process being achieved only with antibiotics. Other typical syndromes of tertiary Lyme borreliosis besides progressive *Borrelia* encephalomyelitis are chronic

Lyme arthritis and acrodermatitis chronica atrophicans. In all three cases *Borrelia* can be detected.

Whereas the acute inflammatory, edematous stage of ACA responds well to antibiotic treatment, the cure is often inadequate if treatment is not commenced until the chronic-atrophic stage. No systematic treatment studies have been carried out. Decades of experience have shown oral and intravenous penicillins or tetracyclines to be effective in principle, though sufficient antibiotic concentrations are only reliably achieved in the skin. This explains the unfavorable courses observed in individual cases. It is therefore advisable, particularly where polyneuritis and/or arthritis are also present, to opt for intravenous treatment with a third-generation cephalosporin over 3 weeks. The same applies where chronic arthritis is present on its own. In the USA up to 10 % of the acute arthritis cases follow a chronic course. Patients who are HLA-DR4-positive are particularly likely to respond poorly to antibiotics. After 3 weeks of antibiotic therapy patients can also be given intraarticular steroids, with synovectomy a last resort in individual cases.

7.1.1.2.4. Therapy during pregnancy

Transplacental passage of *B. burgdorferi* is possible. A causal connection has been well established in individual cases between maternal infection, malformation or death of the child, and detection of *Borrelia* in the fetus. It is not possible to define a typical malformation syndrome. The lack of sufficient data means that the actual frequency of transmission can only be estimated, but it is probably very low. In an American study of 463 newborn babies no connection could be established between the frequency of antibody titers in cord blood and congenital malformation. For the fetus to become infected, the bacterium must be present in the mother's bloodstream. The likelihood of this is greatest at the end of stage I, while erythema migrans is present. In later stages of the disease bacteremia is certainly rare, which means a lower risk. In the light of the isolated reports of congenital malformations despite the mother having been given oral penicillin or erythromycin, intravenous treatment would appear to be a better option. In a Slovenian study of 58 pregnant women with EM there were no complications in 96.6 % of cases, with 5 premature births, 1 abortion, and 1 case of congenital malformation.

In none of these cases was it possible to establish an unequivocal connection with the *Borrelia* infection.

In the majority of cases treatment consisted of ceftriaxone for 14 days (2 g daily). Since this is the only systematic study, it seems advisable to continue with this approach. Cefotaxime is likely to be similarly effective.

7.1.1.2.5. Assessment of the therapeutic outcome

The therapeutic outcome is most effectively assessed on the basis of the clinical symptoms. What is important here is knowledge of the rapidity of the response in individual syndromes. Recommendations for monitoring the treatment of the commonest syndromes are outlined in Tables 7.4-7.7.

Stage I - E(C)M		
Monitoring of treatment	Time:	After 2 and 4 weeks, and after 3 months
	Surrogate markers:	Clinical findings. PCR in urine questionable, serology and general laboratory parameters not prognostically useful.
Course	Complete remission within 4 weeks.	
Prognosis	Treatment failure:	1-3 %
	Delayed cure:	10-23 %
Indication for further treatment	EM not completely gone within 4 weeks, development of new symptoms of stage II	
Strategy	Second 2-week treatment cycle with the same or alternative antibiotic	

Table 7.4: Monitoring of treatment, prognosis, and alternative therapeutic strategies for patients with E[C]M

Whereas EM generally disappears within days, a slow regression of articular pain and swelling is not a sign of treatment failure. The same applies to neuroborreliosis. Radicular pains respond quickly, pareses show only a slow tendency to improve. In the first 7 days there may be some deterioration, which should not prompt a change of treatment.

> As a general rule: the longer the symptom present prior to treatment, the longer it will take to clear, with a distinct increase in likelihood of incomplete cure.

Intravenous antibiotic treatment can trigger a Jarisch-Herxheimer reaction in rare cases. Supplementary steroids given prophylactically may then be beneficial, with continuation of antibiotic treatment.

Inflammatory changes in blood, although present, are not dramatic enough to serve as markers for monitoring treatment. What is of value in neuroborreliosis is repeated testing of the cerebrospinal fluid; the cell count must return to normal within 6 months at most. Slight increases in protein concentrations or in immunoglobulin synthesis may persist for several years and are no cause for concern. No comparable studies of synovial fluid have been carried out. Specific antibodies are poor surrogate markers for monitoring treatment.

Stage II — Neuroborreliosis		
Monitoring of treatment	Time:	2 weeks and 3, 6, and 12 months
	Surrogate marker:	Clinical findings. CSF should be monitored until the cell count returns to normal. Serology not prognostically useful.
Course	Complete remission of the pain symptoms within 10 days. Steady remission of the neurological deficit over the first 3 months, initial deterioration possible, complete remission still possible after a year. Cell count should return to normal within 6 months. Disruption of blood-CSF barrier and intrathecal Ig synthesis may persist as a "CSF scar".	
Prognosis	Treatment failure:	0-3 %
	Delayed cure:	17-33 %
	Incomplete cure:	6-38 %
Indication for further treatment	Pain symptoms persisting more than 2 weeks after therapy, unchanged neurological deficit and persisting pleocytosis over more than 6 months.	
Strategy	Second 3-week treatment cycle. Interval or pulse therapy with cefotaxime can be tried.	

Table 7.5: Monitoring of treatment, prognosis, and alternative therapeutic strategies for patients with neuroborreliosis in stage II

Stage II — Lyme arthritis		
Monitoring of treatment	Time:	2 weeks and 3, 6, and 12 months
	Surrogate marker:	Clinical findings. General laboratory parameters and serology not prognostically useful. Significance of the synovial fluid unknown.
Course	Slow remission of pain and articular effusion within 3 months.	
Prognosis	Treatment failure:	approx. 10 %
	Delayed cure:	approx. 35 %
	Incomplete cure:	unknown
Indication for further treatment	No partial remission within first 4 weeks, articular effusion persisting after 3 months.	
Strategy	If oral therapy given initially, a further 3-week cycle of intravenous antibiotics. Interval or pulse therapy with cefotaxime.	

Table 7.6: Monitoring of treatment, prognosis, and alternative therapeutic strategies for patients with Lyme arthritis in stage II

Stage III — Neuroborreliosis, Lyme arthritis		
Monitoring of treatment	☞ Stage II	
Course	Lyme arthritis:	Very slow remission over one year
	Neuroborreliosis:	Very slow steady remission over up to 3 years. Very slow regression of pleocytosis within 6 months. Disruption of blood-CSF barrier and intrathecal Ig synthesis very often persist as a "CSF scar".
Prognosis	Treatment failure:	unknown
	Delayed cure:	unknown
	Incomplete cure:	*Neuroborreliosis:* 67-100 % *Lyme arthritis:* very common, no numerical data available
Indication for further treatment		*Lyme arthritis:* No partial remission within first 3 months, articular effusion persisting after 3 months *Neuroborreliosis:* Unchanged neurological deficit and pleocytosis persisting more than 6 months after treatment
Strategy		Strategy: ☞ Stage II, plus (Lyme arthritis): synovectomy and/or oral or intraarticular steroids (only after antibiotic treatment).

Table 7.7: Monitoring of treatment, prognosis, and alternative therapeutic strategies for patients with neuroborreliosis and Lyme arthritis in stage III

Even after a successful course of antibiotic treatment elevated antibody titers may still be present. Persistence for years, even of IgM antibodies, is known to occur in all three stages of the disease. The decline of the antibody concentration over years varies greatly from one individual to the next, and it is therefore pointless monitoring the course of the antibodies in the short term. Proof of seronegativity can, however, be useful if reinfection is suspected.

Direct detection of the pathogen by culture or by PCR is more suitable as a means of therapeutic monitoring. Culture of Borrelia from body fluids and tissues is laborious and only comes into question in scientific studies. The drawback of PCR is its low sensitivity (approx. 30 %) in CSF and urine. If, however, a positive result is obtained after antibiotic treatment has been completed, this can be very useful therapeutically, particularly when striving to differentiate between clinical deficit symptoms and persisting inflammation. This has been well established in smaller patient populations. The testing can be carried out on urine, CSF, or the synovial fluid.

7.1.2. Prognosis, relapse, treatment resistance, and delayed cure

The prognosis (☞ Tables 7.4-7.7) in Lyme borreliosis must be classified as very favorable if adequate treatment appropriate to the stage and the syndrome is given. Resistance to treatment can be expected to occur in a mere handful of cases in stages I and II. Delayed cures appear to be more common in stage III, and include patients whose clinical symptoms take longer than average to recede, most of these being patients in whom deficits continue to persist. The incidence of incomplete cures in neuroborreliosis ranges from 6 to 38 % in stage II and is up to 100 % in stage III. The available data relating to resistance to treatment in stage III are ambiguous. Whereas in the American literature this is reported in up to 70 % of Lyme arthritis patients, in Europe it is expected to occur in only a few percent of the cases.

> It is therefore always advisable to assess the diagnosis critically before assuming resistance to treatment.

What is unclear is whether an endogenous relapse can occur after complete regression of the symptoms. The cases that have been described are most likely to have been reinfections or secondary conditions unrelated to the borreliosis. In cases of resistance to treatment and delayed cure a further treatment cycle was effective. After the treatment Borrelia was subsequently isolated from the CSF, synovial fluid, skin, and the heart valves, so that persistence of the pathogen must clearly be held responsible for the poorer prognosis in individual cases. Regular checkups should therefore be given at 3-monthly intervals for up to a year in stages II and III. Should the question of a further treatment cycle arise, there are various approaches of unproven efficacy based on theories concerning the pathophysiology of Lyme borreliosis. Strategies that have been proposed include longer treatment periods, higher doses, and pulse or interval therapy. Pragmatically, a second 3-week cycle of intravenous treatment with a third-generation cephalosporin (e.g. cefotaxime or ceftriaxone) can be tried first. The antibiotic must not be changed, since secondary antibiotic resistance has never been reported. Alternatively, cases have been described in which patients were successfully given high-dose cefotaxime 3 × 4 g on 2 consecutive days followed by 5 days without treatment, with a total of 6-8 such cycles (pulse therapy; ☞ Table 7.8).

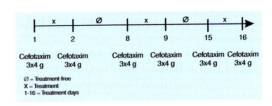

Table 7.8: Regimen for pulse therapy in treatment-refractory cases (6-8 cycles)

This treatment regimen is based on the theoretical consideration that tissues with a poor blood supply are likely to be good sites for *Borrelia* persistence. Only by using extremely high antibiotic concentrations is it possible in such cases to eradicate *Borrelia*. A further consideration, in view of the long generation time of *Borrelia* and the development of persister forms, is that it might be beneficial to include treatment-free intervals in the course of the treatment. Despite the lack of data on this innovative regimen, it might make sense to attempt pulse therapy in treatment-refractory cases. The alternative is pure interval therapy. This concept is currently under investigation by our own research group within the framework of a multicenter study, with particular emphasis on whether such an approach could be superior to conventional long-term treatment already in the primary treatment of neuroborreliosis (CEFBO study, cefotaxime 3 × 2 g for 19 days versus 1 week of 3 × 2 g daily, followed by 3-day periods of 3 × 2 g alternating with 3 days without treatment). Successful treatment by immunomodulation with recombinant interleukin-4 and anti-interleukin-12 antibodies has been reported in experimental animal studies, but has not been investigated in humans.

7.2. Tick-borne encephalitis (TBE)

7.2.1. Therapy

In the case of TBE there is no causal therapy. Virostatics effective against other viral infections are not reliably beneficial. The same applies to amantadine, which is occasionally recommended.

> Immunoglobulins are not indicated at any time in the manifest stage of the disease, either in the form of a hyperimmune serum or as polyvalent preparations.

In the cases reported in the literature such treatment has not been found to offer any benefit to the patient. At a dose of 0.4 g/kg i.v. for 5 days, as is administered in certain neuroimmunological conditions, an unfavorable effect on the endogenous neutralizing antibodies production must even be feared, owing to the immunomodulating action of immunoglobulins and autoregulation of the immune system. There is likewise no indication for glucocorticoids. The success of treatment with hydrocortisone reported in 1975 by Duniewicz was based on individual experience and was not controlled by clinical studies.

Because of the possibility of bacterial meningitis, which cannot be ruled out initially on the basis of CSF findings, antibiotic treatment, e.g. with cefotaxime 2 × 2 g/day and ampicillin 3 × 2 g/day (owing to the possibility of listeriosis), is recommended until serological confirmation of acute TBE infection has been obtained.

Treatment of TBE
• Parenteral fluids
• Analgesia
• Thrombosis prophylaxis
• Anticonvulsant treatment in the event of attacks

Table 7.9: Treatment of TBE

Treatment of TBE is limited to symptomatic measures (☞ Table 7.9). In most cases parenteral fluids are required on account of the high fever and lethargy. Analgesia is necessary for severe headaches and for segmental pains within the framework of myelitis and radiculitis. Simple analgesics such as paracetamol, acetylsalicylic acid, or diclofenac are often insufficiently effective. Our own experience has shown metamizol (Novalgin®) to be highly beneficial to patients on a temporary basis at least. *Temporary* anticonvulsant prophylaxis is only necessary if attacks have already occurred.

7.2.2. Prognosis

The long-term prognosis in TBE is often less favorable than in other viral infections of the nervous system. The intensity of the symptoms during the acute phase of the disease correlates to some degree with the nature and duration of the complaints during the convalescence phase. In the first large review of TBE Duniewicz reported a renewed worsening of the disease in 50 % of his patients at the first follow-up examination, with symptoms such as headaches, tiredness, sleep disturbances, and often dizziness and increased irritability. However, Duniewicz did not state how many patients had been followed up for acute illness, and at what intervals this had taken place. The objective findings reported were tremor of the fingers and eyelids, atactic disturbances, and, more rarely, nystagmus. At the second follow-up examination only a quarter of the patients were still unfit for work. The total duration of time off work after discharge from hospital was 6-10 weeks, and around 10 % of the patients continued to report subjective symptoms such as frequent tiredness, headaches, and sleep disturbances after returning to work. Individual patients suffered from depression, requiring specialist medical treatment. In a later study of 299 patients, by Ackermann et al., the cure was delayed in 14 % of the cases and was incomplete in a further 7 %. Similar statistics have been reported by Köck et al. in a follow-up study of 117 TBE patients: Discrete subjective individual symptoms were observed in 13 % of the cases and appreciable physical incapacitation in 5 %. Most individual case studies that have been published describe relatively serious clinical courses for TBE, with correspondingly long convalescence phases and neurological deficits.

In more than 500 cases reported since 1994 in Baden-Württemberg intensive-care treatment was necessary in 14 % of the cases and assisted ventilation in 5 %. On discharge 20 % of the patients still had temporary deficits (lasting up to 6 months) such as a pronounced neurasthenic syndrome, co-ordination disturbances, tremor of the extremities, mono- and hemipareses, and concentration and memory disturbances, and 10 % had persistent neurological deficits such as hypoacusis, coordination disturbances, pareses, or a respiratory failure requiring assisted ventilation. In 16 % of patients further rehabilitation measures were necessary after the acute treatment.

Hypoacusis as a symptom of TBE was previously reported only by Duniewicz. Although hearing disturbances and vestibular dizziness have frequently been mentioned as individual complaints after TBE, we have never observed the simultaneous occurrence of both complaints in our own follow-up studies. Pareses of the oculomotor nerves and of the facial nerve were only short-lived, both in the study of Duniewicz and in our own work. In the patient population studied by Duniewicz pareses of the caudal cranial nerves were found to recede rapidly, whereas in 6 patients with meningoencephalomyelitis whom we monitored the function of these cranial nerves did not recover over the next 5 years or until death.

The tendency of pareses of the extremities to regress correlates well with the extent and rate of development of the initial symptoms. The regression is substantially slower in myelitis than in radiculitis. Early onset of severe pareses accompanied by respiratory paralysis is generally associated with a poor prognosis. Lethal outcomes in TBE are seen above all in patients who developed quadriparesis and respiratory failure within 1-3 days of the onset of the second febrile phase. Mild pareses, on the other hand, may regress completely within a few weeks or months.

In most cases the general changes in the EEG often observed during the acute phase of the disease recede within a few weeks or months. Focal changes in the EEG nearly always show a distinct tendency to regress, though in patients with severe forms of the disease they are sometimes still discernible more than one year later. In our own studies epileptic fits were never encountered after the end of the acute phase.

The **lethality** of the disease was reported in the 1960s and 1970s to be between 3 and 5 %. More recent studies show this figure to have fallen to some 1-2 %.

References

Ackermann R., Kruger K., Roggendorf M., Rehse-Kupper B., Mortter M., Schneider M. (1986). Vukadinovic I: Spread of early-summer meningo-encephalitis in the Federal Republic of Germany. Dtsch. Med. Wschr. 111: 927-933

Ackermann R., Rehse-Kupper B. (1979). Die Zentraleuropäische Enzephalitis in der Bundesrepublik Deutschland. Fortschr. Neurol. Psychiat. 47: 103-122

Blumenthal W., Ackermann R., Schottky A. (1970). Zentraleuropäische Enzephalitis unter dem Bild einer lumbalen Poliomyelitis. Med. Klinik 65: 153-156

Bodemann H., Pausch J., Schmitz H., Hoppe-Seyler P. (1977). Die Zeckenenzephalitis (FSME) als Labor-Infektion. Med. Welt. 28: 1779-1781

Dattwyler R.J., Halperin J.J., Volkman D.J., Luft B.J. (1988). Treatment of late Lyme borreliosis - randomised comparison of ceftriaxone and penicillin. Lancet II: 1191-1194

Duniewicz M. (1976). Klinisches Bild der Zentraleuropäischen Zeckenenzephalitis. Münch. Med. Wschr. 118: 1609-1612

Gunther G., Haglund M., Lindquist L., Forsgren M., Skoldenberg B. (1997). Tick-bone encephalitis in Sweden in relation to aseptic meningo-encephalitis of other etiology: a prospective study of clinical course and outcome. J. Neurol. 244: 230-238

Haglund M., Forsgren M., Lindh G., Lindquist L. (1996). A 10-year follow-up study of tick-borne encephalitis in the Stockholm area and a review of the literature: need for a vaccination strategy. Scand. J. Infect. Dis. 28: 217-224

Hammers-Berggren S., Lebech A.M., Karlsson M., Svenungsson B., Hansen K., Stiernstedt G. (1994). Serological follow-up after treatment of patients with erythema migrans and neuroborreliosis. J. Clin. Microbiol. 32: 1519-1525

Hassler D., Zöller L., Haude M., Hufnagel H.D., Heinrich F., Sonntag H.G. (1990). Cefotaxime versus penicillin in the late stage of Lyme disease - prospective, randomized therapeutic study. Infection 18: 16-20

Kaiser R., Braun H., Dörstelmann D., Hansmann P., von Laer D., Lücking C.H, Wagner K. (1996). Die Frühsommer-Meningoenzephalitis - Beobachtungen zur Klinik und Häufigkeit im Schwarzwald 1994. Akt. Neurologie 23: 21-25

Kaiser R., Vollmer H., Schmidtke K., Rauer S., Berger W., Gores D. (1997). Follow-up and prognosis of early summer meningoencephalitis. Nervenarzt 68: 324-330

Karlsson M., Hammers-Berggren S., Lindquist L., Stiernstedt G., Svenungsson B. (1994). Comparison of intravenous penicillin G and oral doxycycline for treatment of Lyme neuroborreliosis. Neurology 44: 1203-1207

Kock T., Stunzner D., Freidl W., Pierer K. (1992). Clinical aspects of early summer meningoencephalitis in Styria. Nervenarzt 63: 205-208

Kohlhepp W., Oschmann P., Mertens H.G. (1989). Treatment of Lyme borreliosis. Randomized comparison of doxycycline and penicillin G. J. Neuro. 236: 464-469

Kramer M.D., Hassler D., Hofmann H., Wallich R., Schaible U.E., Simon M.M. (1993). Therapie der Lyme-Borreliose. Dtsch. Med. Wschr. 118: 469-473

Krüger H., Reuss K., Pulz M., Rohrbach E., Pflughaupt K.W., Martin R., Mertens H.G. (1989). Meningoradiculitis and encephalomyelitis due to *Borrelia burgdorferi*: a follow-up study of 72 patients over 27 years. J. Neurol. 236: 322-328

Maraspin V., Cimperman J., Lotric-Furlan S., Pleterski-Rigler D., Strle F. (1996). Treatment of Erythema Migrans in Pregnancy. Clinical Infectious Diseases 22: 788-793

Oschmann P., Dorndorf W. (1995). Therapie der Lyme-Borreliose. Versicherungsmedizin 47: 79-83

Pfister H.W., Preac-Mursic V., Einhäupl K.M., Wilske B. (1989). Cefotaxime versus penicillin G for acute neurological manifestations of Lyme borreliosis: a prospective randomized study. Arch. Neurol. 46: 1190-1194

Pfister H.W., Preac-Mursic V., Wilske B., Schielke E., Soergel F., Einhäupl K.M. (1991). Randomized comparison of ceftriaxone and cefotaxime in Lyme neuroborreliosis. J. Infect. Dis. 163: 311-318

Sigal L.H. (1995). Management of Lyme Disease Refractory to Antibiotic Therapy. Rheumatic Disease Clinica of North America 21: 217-230

Stiernstedt G. (1993). Therapeutic Aspects of Lyme Borreliosis. Clinics in Dermatology 11: 423-429

Weber K., Preac-Mursic V., Wilske B., Thurmayr R., Neubert U., Scherwitz C. (1990). A randomized trial of ceftriaxone versus oral penicillin for treatment of early Lyme borreliosis. Infection 18: 91-96

Prophylactic measures

8. Prophylactic measures

8.1. General protection measures

In contrast to spring-summer encephalitis, for Lyme borreliosis there are still no options available in Europe for active or passive immunization.

> Registration of a monovalent borreliosis vaccine is expected imminently in the USA. However, the heterogeneity of the various *Borrelia* serotypes means that its efficacy in Europe is none too certain.

Consequently, measures aimed at protection against tick bites constitute the first line of defense in prophylaxis of Lyme borreliosis. By observing such precautions the risk of TBE infection can be reduced, even in the regions where the disease is endemic.

8.1.1. General protection against ticks

The risk of infection can be substantially reduced by avoiding habitats with a high tick density, such as wooded areas with luxuriant undergrowth and dense vegetation (e.g. bracken or broom). Ticks can also be passed on directly by domestic and wild animals. This is possible so long as the ticks are not yet firmly attached to the host animal. It is therefore important to inspect cats and dogs living alongside humans regularly for ticks. In handling freshly bagged game animals, which are often massively tick-infested, hunters should take care to avoid picking up ticks when transporting and breaking up the carcasses. Not only precautionary measures but also suitable clothing play an appreciable role in tick protection. After transferring to a human, ticks are quite capable of crawling around clothing for hours at a time until they find an area of bare skin. It is therefore important to wear tightly fitting clothing with long sleeves and trousers. Insect repellants (e.g. diethyltoluamide, Autan®) can also be sprayed onto clothes. After venturing into tick habitats it is advisable to check the whole body and clothing for ticks.

8.1.2. Removal of ticks

Even after discovering a firmly attached tick it is still possible to reduce the risk of infection. Each tick should be removed immediately upon discovery.

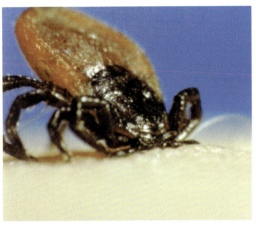

a

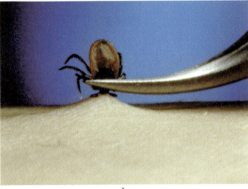

b

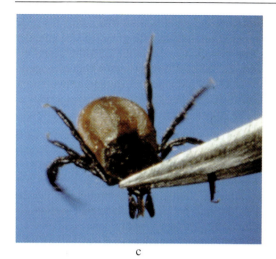

Figs. 8.1a-c: **a**: Female Ixodes ricinus, not long after attachment to a human host. **b**: Removal of the attached female Ixodes ricinus with tweezers. **c**: Female Ixodes ricinus after complete removal (with the kind permission of Prof. Matuschka, Inst. of Pathology, Charité, Berlin)

The risk of transmission depends largely on the length of time the tick has been sucking. Experiments show that *Borrelia* infection does not occur until at least 12 h (and in many cases not until some 72 h) after commencement of sucking. The method by which the tick is removed may also make a difference: squeezing of the tick must always be avoided so as not to expel any *Borreliae* present in the gut into the host organism.

> The safest way to remove a tick is with a pair of tweezers (☞ Fig. 8.1b), holding the tweezers as close as possible to the point of attachment. Slight twisting and pulling movements loosen the grip of the mouthparts, allowing the removal of the tick (☞ Fig. 8.1c).

If the head breaks off and remains in the skin, a local foreign body reaction can develop. The risk of a *Borrelia* infection will be low in such cases, as the bacterium lives in the tick's body (mainly in the midgut). Like any other foreign object (e.g. a splinter) the head should be removed from the skin and the point of entry disinfected. It is possible to test removed ticks for *Borrelia*, though it has not yet been confirmed that this makes sense in principle as the basis for any subsequent antibiotic treatment.

8.1.3. Tick control

In addition to personal protective measures, a reduction in the risk of infection can be achieved by direct tick control. One option is the ecologically highly questionable destruction of the tick's habitat. In the USA, through clearing, mowing, and burning of vegetation the adult tick population was reduced by some 70-88 %, though the fall in numbers lasted no longer than a year. In gardens and parks fallen leaves are a good habitat, and their regular removal is therefore recommended. One alternative that has been attempted is application of insecticides to problem areas. This was not very effective, as ticks spend most of their life buried in the soil. A high density of host animals is also known to bring substantial tick densities in its wake. This is particularly true where wild animals are present in large numbers in a closely confined area. Regulated wildlife stock control can thus be an important factor. Attempts have also been made to reduce the tick infestation of host animals. In the USA the white-footed mouse (*Peromyscus locpus*) serves as an important reservoir for *B. burgdorferi*. In affected areas wads of cotton wool soaked with the insect repellent permethrin were left in mouse habitats. The white-footed mice used the cotton wool as welcome nesting material, thereby treating themselves against ticks. Follow-up investigations showed 72 % of mice to be tick-free. A similar result can be achieved with domestic animals by the use of insecticide-treated collars.

8.2. Lyme borreliosis

In contrast to TBE, passive or active immunization following a tick bite is not possible in the case of Lyme borreliosis. Prophylactic antibiotic treatment is conceivable after being bitten, but is not recommended in view of the low risk of contracting Lyme borreliosis (approx. 1-5 %) and the very good response to antibiotics in early stages of the disease. A sensible approach is to tell the patients about the relative risks and benefits of prophylactic treatment, and to explain the possible symptoms of illness. In individual cases, e.g. patients who are very anxious, a serological test can be performed immediately after the bite to establish seronegativity (baseline value) and again 2 and 4 weeks later. If seroconversion is subsequently demonstrated, the patient can undergo a cycle of treatment. However, the presence of antibodies does not necessarily mean that the disease will develop. This has been shown to occur only in about 1 case in 6. Pregnant women should always undergo serological monitoring after a tick bite, as it is not yet known for certain how high is the actual risk of damage to the fetus after a *Borrelia* infection. The indication for treatment should be interpreted very generously in such cases.

Vaccine development

Johnson in 1986 was the first to show in an animal model (mice) that active immunization with a "whole cell preparation" offered protection against *B. burgdorferi*. Two vaccine products based on inactivated *Borreliae* have been registered in the USA for the treatment of dogs. No such products have been registered for humans, owing to fears that an immunological reaction against host antigens might be triggered, as *Borreliae* possess epitopes cross-reacting with human cells. In the hamster model a destructive arthritis could be triggered after inoculation with a whole-cell vaccine.

A safe option has proved to be preparations of surface proteins (☞ Section 2.1.5.). In an animal model protection was achieved by injections of recombinant OspA, OspB and OspC, and OspF, the degree of efficacy being dependent on the immunogen used. Use of recombinant OspE afforded no protection at all. The best studied is the OspA vaccine. The Freiburg research group of the Max-Planck Institute for Immunobiology (*Dr. Simon*) in particular has shown that both active and passive immunization with OspA as the immunogen results in complete protection in mice. Immunization either with recombinant lipidated OspA or with plasmid-DNA that codes for OspA was shown to stimulate specific B-cell and T-cell responses and adequate concentrations of protective antibodies. In experimental studies in mice the best protection against infection was achieved when the protective antibodies were already present prior to the infection. This is probably due to the action mechanism of OspA-specific antibodies, which already begin to eradicate the spirochetes inside the tick if ingested during sucking (cf. Section 2.1.4.). One problem has proved to be the heterogeneity of the OspA-proteins in different isolates (cf. Section 2.1.5.). There is little or no protection against infections with a *Borrelia* strain whose OspA-protein differs from the recombinant OspA protein injected. In the USA this seems unlikely to be a problem, owing the high homogeneity of OspA serotypes. In Europe a monovalent OspA vaccine may prove ineffective as a result of the heterogeneity of *Borrelia* serotypes.

Two monovalent recombinant **OspA vaccines** have been developed by Pasteur Merieux Connaught and by SmithKline Beecham, and have proved reliable in phase I and II studies in the USA. In a double-blind placebo-controlled multicenter phase III study of 10 306 volunteers completed in March 1996 (Pasteur Merieux Connaught) the vaccine was shown to be effective at least in the USA.

- Volunteers were given three injections of either the OspA vaccine (ImuLyme) or placebo at time-points 0, 1, and 12 months
- Efficacy was age- and sex-dependent
- After two injections the vaccine was 89 % effective in men under 60, but not in those above this age limit
- Corresponding efficacy in women was 67 % (below 60) and 47 % (over 60)
- After three injections efficacy in men rose to 100 % (below 60) and 67 % (over 60)
- For women 100 % efficacy was observed after the third vaccination, this being independent of age

Side effects were few and comprised slight reddening and swelling at the site of injection. The actively treated group also complained more often of chills, muscle pains, and headaches. A disappointment was the duration of the vaccine protection, observed in a smaller study on 83 volunteers. After primary immunization all volunteers developed antibodies against OspA, but with one exception these were no longer detectable 180 days later. Furthermore, in cell cultures the antibodies were found to afford protection only against the strain used in the vaccine itself, and not against other strains of *Borrelia*. No other data have been published so far on this problem. In the meantime the first results have also been published from a second double-blind placebo-controlled multicenter phase III study of the competing SmithKline Beecham vaccine. In this study 10 936 participants, all American, were given three injections of the L-Osp-A vaccine (plus aluminum as adjuvant) or placebo in a 0, 1, and 12 months vaccination regimen. In the actively treated group there were 13 cases of Lyme borreliosis, compared with 61 in the placebo group (p = 0.0001). The efficacy was 79 % after three injections and 50 % after two. Side effects were few. Still unclarified (or else not yet published) is how long the vaccine protection lasts and how soon booster doses are required.

As mentioned at the beginning, for European conditions these vaccines must be modified in order to afford protection against serotypes of all three genospecies that are pathogenic to humans — *B. burgdorferi* sensu strictu, *Borrelia afzelii*, and *Borrelia garinii*. Because of these difficulties the suitability of other materials as antigen candidates for vaccines is currently being investigated in animal models. The furthest advanced of these is the development of OspC vaccines. Investigations of proteins important to the dissemination of *Borreliae* in tissue (decorin-binding protein and plasminogen-binding protein) are in an early experimental stage.

8.3. Tick-borne encephalitis

In view of the clinical situation described, prophylactic *active vaccination* is recommended for persons likely to be exposed in high-risk areas. Two such vaccines are available: Encepur® (Chiron Behring) and TBE-Immun® (Immuno). The vaccines consist of the complete inactivated virion. The vaccine virus is propagated on chick embryo fibroblasts, highly purified by various centrifugation steps, and finally inactivated. Prior to release all batches of the vaccine are tested for viable viruses by intracerebral inoculation of newborn white mice. Both vaccines are highly immunogenic and achieve a seroconversion rate of > 95 % after only the second immunization.

To ensure adequate vaccine protection up to the onset of seasonal tick activity, the recommended option is active vaccination during the winter months according to the so-called long-term regimen, though this can also be done at any time during the year.

TBE long-term regimen (Chiron Behring, Baxter-Immuno)	
1st injection	day 0
2nd injection	after 1-2 months
3rd injection	after 9-12 months
Booster immunizations	after 3 years

Table 8.1: TBE-prophylaxis: long-term regimen.

TBE fast immunization (Chiron Behring)	
1st injection	day 0
2nd injection	day 7
3rd injection	day 21
4th injection	after 12-18 months
Booster immunizations	after 3 years

Table 8.2: TBE-prophylaxis: fast immunization

Basic immunization by the long-term regimen consists of three partial immunizations (☞ Table 8.1). Because many people decide to be immunized only at the last minute at the start of the tick season, there is considerable interest in a regimen with which vaccine protection is built up as quickly as possible. This goal is achieved with the so-called **fast immunization** (☞ Table 8.2). In the study with the Chiron-Behring product (N = 379 volunteers) the neutralization test demonstrated a seroconversion rate of > 99 % as soon as two weeks after the second immunization (i.e. on day 21). With the Immuno product too vaccine protection can be built up more quickly by shortening the interval between the first and second inoculations to 10 days, though this is based on only one small study of 37 children immunized twice with an interval of 10 days. In this study immunization was shown to have taken hold after 14 days in 34 of the 37 children (92 %), as evidenced by a positive hemagglutination-inhibition test. To complete the basic immunization, a further booster is necessary after 12-18 months.

Further booster doses after 3-5 years are recommended. In the absence of published data on the frequency and duration of the often longer-lasting vaccine protection in some individuals, but also in view of some individuals contracting TBE 4 years after their last immunization, a more advisable option is a further booster dose either 3 years after the last immunization or according to the antibody status. The vaccine is best given by an intramuscular injection, and owing to the unreliable absorption into fatty tissue in overweight people it should be given into the deltoid muscle rather than the buttocks.

The cascade of events triggered in the organism by the immunogens and other constituents present in the vaccine leads to various reactions, some of them desirable and some not so. A distinction must be made here between vaccine reactions (side effects) and vaccine complications (vaccine damage and vaccine failure). Both the immunizing agent itself and the excipients (preserving agents and stabilizers) present in the vaccine products must be considered as possible triggers for **vaccine reactions**. In an analysis of 595 **spontaneously reported suspected cases** of vaccine side effects of the Chiron-Behring product, the most frequent reaction in all groups was slight fever of up to 39°C, the next commonest being generalized reactions with headaches, fatigue, and occasionally vomiting. In one case, fever in an 18-month-old boy resulted in a fit of convulsions.

On the basis of clinical studies a different distribution frequency must be assumed for vaccine reactions: local reactions (pain, swelling, and/or reddening at the site of injection) must be expected in up to 20 % of the cases, headaches in 5-28 %, and generalized reactions (fatigue, limb pains) in 7-13 %. Vaccine reactions such as these occur in over 90 % of the cases after the first vaccination against TBE, and are only rarely seen after subsequent doses. In most cases these vaccine reactions subside within 1-3 days and have no lasting consequences.

In comparison with vaccine reactions, **vaccine complications** after TBE vaccination are very rare. In the period between 1971 and 1990 there was just one single acknowledged case of vaccine damage (40 % reduction in fitness for work) after active TBE vaccination. According to a communiqué issued by the Drug Committee of the German medical profession a total of 528 suspected cases of adverse drug reactions (ADRs) after TBE vaccination were reported between 1985 and 1993. In 224 of these cases the symptoms concerned the central and peripheral nervous system. Since in many cases insufficient information was available for an assessment to be made, it was only possible to analyse 92 of these suspected cases. Only in 2 of them was the connection between the neurological symptoms (neuritis) and the earlier vaccination assessed as certain, and in 3 other cases it was viewed as probable. In view of this assessment and the number of vaccine doses sold, the risk of vaccine complications in TBE is estimated at about one in a million vaccinations.

Whereas this assessment was based on the Venulet recommendations, more recent American guidelines specify stricter criteria for assessing the connection between an ADR and a vaccination. In particular, demonstration of a causal connection is required to attribute an ADR to a vaccination. For assessing the probability of the connection between an ADR and a prior vaccination, the Vaccine Safety Committee of the Institute of Medicine lists five categories:

- **1:** *No evidence* of any causal connection
- **2:** The data are *insufficient* for accepting or rejecting the connection
- **3:** The data suggest *the absence of a causal connection*
- **4:** The data suggest *the presence of a causal connection*
- **5:** The data *confirm the connection*

This classification is based on weighted published data and on biological plausibilities. As far as the published data on vaccine complications are concerned, least value is attached to individual case reports and most to placebo-controlled prospective studies. Of special importance too is the time window within which an ADR can be credibly (with biological plausibility) attributed to a vaccination on the basis of experimental animal data and clinical findings. The period between the 7th and 21st day after vaccination can be regarded as typical and the period between the 5th and the 42nd days as the maximum plausible interval between vaccination and onset of neurological complications.

Taking account of these recommendations, an analysis has been carried out of all suspected cases of ADRs after active TBE vaccination published between 1980 and 1996. In 9 out of the 16 cases the ADR was within the plausible time interval. In 7 of these 9 patients the clinical symptoms (myelitis, polyradiculitis, neuritis, ataxia, myalgias, mutism, vestibulopathy) subsided completely within 2-120 days, persistence of the acute neurological symptoms (vestibulopathy, myelitis) being reported in only 2 cases. In the myelitis patient considerable doubt has since been cast by the assessor on the causal connection between vaccination and the neurological symptoms. Summarizing, it is not possible to deduce any typical pattern of neurological damage after TBE vaccination on the basis of the published cases.

The "arznei-telegramm" communication identifying multiple sclerosis as a consequence of vaccine damage after TBE vaccination was not confirmed by our own research at the National Office for the Disabled in Vienna. In the case cited it was the triggering not of the disease itself but of a relapse that was recognized as a consequence of vaccination. However, other findings suggest that the risk of triggering a relapse in MS patients by a vaccination is no greater than could be expected from the individual relapse rate. The need for thorough differential-diagnostic clarification where vaccine complications are suspected has been emphasized by Wiersbitzky et al.: An etiology other than vaccination was established as the cause of the clinical symptoms in all 58 cases of suspected ADRs they investigated. Because of a certain instinctive need to establish causality, where the vaccination has been given to protect the central nervous system against infection there may be a tendency to interpret any CNS disturbances in particular as vaccine complications. However, since the TBE vaccination uses a killed vaccine whose safety is tested in animals for every batch, infection of the nervous system due to the vaccine can be ruled out. Thus, in theory, since only toxic and immunological damage is conceivable, there is no reason at all why this should be confined to the nervous system and in principle it could affect any bodily system.

Administration of specific immunoglobulins has proved beneficial in certain infectious diseases (tetanus, diphtheria, rabies, hepatitis B, cytomegalovirus and varicella zoster infection), the efficacy of this being determined essentially by a sufficiently high dose and by a suitably short interval between the infection date and administration of the immunoglobulin. The benefits of administering exogenous specific antibodies (passive immunization) have been demonstrated in the case of TBE in experimental animal studies. The rate of protection with *passive immunization* in humans after tick bite in a high-risk area (post-exposure prophylaxis) was, however, calculated at only some 50-60 % on the basis of survey findings. Since some particularly severe cases of TBE have occurred in children in temporal association with passive immunization, the registration of this indication for children and adolescents up to the age of 14 is currently suspended in accordance with a ruling from the Paul Ehrlich Institute. In this age group TBE is normally overwhelmingly manifested as meningitis with a good prognosis. The connection between severe forms of the disease and passive immunization has yet to be clarified in such cases.

For persons over 14 a dose of 0.2 ml hyperimmunoglobulin per kg is recommended. The interval between the probable onset of infection (entering the endemic zone → tick bite) and the passive immunization should not exceed 48 h. Since some 40 % of patients with manifest TBE do not recall being bitten by a tick, and since the incubation period for TBE can be up to 3 weeks, post-exposure prophylaxis with immunoglobulins after tick bite should not be given to persons who had entered a high-risk area repeatedly in the preceding 3 weeks. Thus, passive immunization does not as a rule constitute adequate prophylaxis of TBE for those living in high-risk areas. In view of the considerably lower costs and distinctly longer-lasting and more reliable protection, inhabitants of high-risk areas should be made increasingly aware of the possibility of active immunization.

So far there is no general recommendation for **simultaneous immunization** (active and passive immunization), such as is given for tetanus. Active immunization immediately after a tick bite also has not been officially recommended up to now. The possibility of this measure has, however, been discussed during a meeting of experts in this field, the purpose of the active immunization being not to prevent illness after a potential infection but to stop future TBE infections from occurring. If TBE does not develop, active immunization must then be completed in accordance with the vaccination plan.

References

Aebi C., Schaad U.B. (1994). TBE-immunoglobulins - a critical assessment of efficacy. Schweiz. Med. Wschr. 124: 1837-1840

Anonymous. (1995). Multiple Sklerose nach FSME-Impfung in Österreich als Impfschädigung anerkannt. Arzneitelegramm 3: 32

Anonymous. (1996). Pressemitteilung des Paul-Ehrlich-Instituts vom 30.08.96. Epidemiologisches Bulletin 36: 249

Arzneimittelkommission der deutschen Ärzteschaft. (1996). Impfung gegen Frühsommer-Meningoenzephalitis: Nutzen - Risiken - Indikation. Ärztebl. Baden-Württemberg 4:142-143

DeNoon D.D. (1996). Lyme Disease (Clinical studies: More bad news for Lyme disease Vaccine. News Reports November 25 & December 2

Fikrig E., Barthold S.W., Kantor F.S., Flavell R.A. (1990). Protection of Mice Against the Lyme Disease Agent by Immunizing with Recombinant OspA. Science 250: 553-556

Gern L., Hu C.M., Voet P., Hauser P., Lobet Y. (1997). Immunization with a polyvalent OspA vaccine protects mice against Ixodes ricinus tick bites infected by *Borrelia burgdorferi* s.s., *Borrelia garinii* and *Borrelia afzelii*. Vaccine 15: 1551-1557

Gold R., Wiethoelter H., Rihs I., Löwer J., Kappos L. (1992). Frühsommer-Meningoenzephalitis-Impfung. Indikation und kritische Beurteilung neurologischer Impfkomplikationen. Dtsch. Med. Wschr. 117: 112-116

Harabacz I., Bock H., Jungst C., Klockmann U., Praus M., Weber R. (1992). A randomized phase II study of a new tick-borne encephalitis vaccine using three different doses and two immunization regimens. Vaccine 10: 145-150

Heinz F.X., Tuma W., Kunz C. (1981). Antigenic and immunogenic properties of defined physical forms of tick-borne encephalitis virus structural proteins. Infection. Immun. 33: 250-257

Hofmann H. (1995). After vaccination for tick-borne encephalitis must onset of neurologic disorders be expected? Wien. Klin. Wschr. 107: 509-515

Kaiser R. (1996). Die FSME in Südwestdeutschland unter besonderer Berücksichtigung der Verläufe im Kindesalter. Hautnah Pädiatrie 3: 186-192

Kaiser R. (1997). FSME-Impfung. Akt. Neurologie 24: 124-128

Kluger G., Waldvogel K. (1995). Tick-borne encephalitis despite specific immunoglobulin prophylaxis. Lancet 346: 1502

Kunz C., Heinz F.X., Hofmann H. (1980). Immunogenicity and reactogenecity of a highly purified vaccine against tick-borne encephalitis. J. Med. Virol. 8: 103-109

Kunz C., Hofmann H., Dippe H. (1991). Early summer meningoencephalitis vaccination, a preventive medicine measure with high acceptance in Austria. Wien. Med. Wschr. 141: 273-276

Kunz C., Hofmann H., Kundi M. (1981). Zur Wirksamkeit von FSME-Immunglobulin. Wien. Klin. Wschr. 93: 665-667

Quast U., Fescharek R., Rosenkranz G. (1993). Verträglichkeit der FSME-Vaccine Behring. Erfahrungen der ersten Impfsaison. Der Kinderarzt 2: 193-199

Quast U., Herder C., Zwisler O. (1991). Vaccination of patients with encephalomyelitis disseminata. Vaccine 9: 228-230

Quast U., Thilo W., Fescharek R. (1993). Impfreaktionen - Bewertung und Differentialdiagnose. Stuttgart, Hippokrates Verlag

Sibley W., Bamford C., Laguna J. (1976). Influenza vaccination in patients with multiple sclerosis. J. Am. Med. Ass. 236: 1965-1966

Stratton K.R., Howe C.J., Johnston R.B. (1994). Causality and evidence. In: Stratton K.R., Howe C.J., Johnston R.B. (eds): 33. Washington, D.C., National Academy Press

Venulet J. (1984). Methoden der Überwachung und Dokumentation unerwünschter Arzneimittelwirkungen. In: Kümmerle-Stitzenberger (ed): Klinische Pharmakologie. Landsberg, Ecomed

Wiersbitzky S., Bruns R., Mentel R. (1993). Verdacht auf Impfkomplikationen oder atypischer Impfverlauf. Diagnostische Abklärung bei 58 Impflingen. Kinderärztl. Praxis 61: 329-334

Wormser G.P. (1997). Treatment and Prevention of Lyme Disease, with Emphasis on Antimicrobial Therapy for Neuroborreliosis and Vaccination. Seminars in Neurology 17: 45-52

Zastrow K., Schöneberg I. (1994). Anerkannte Impfschäden in der Bundesrepublik Deutschland 1971-1990. Bundesgesundheitsblatt 3: 109-112

Zhong W., Ger L., Kramer M., Wallich R., Simon M.M. (1997). T helper cell priming of mice to *Borrelia burgdorferi* OspA leads to induction of protective antibodies following experimental but not tick-borne infection. Eur. J. Immunol. 27: 4942-4947

Zhong W., Stehle T., Museteanu C., Siebers A., Gern L., Kramer M., Wallich R., Simon M.M. (1997). Therapeutic passive vaccination against chronic Lyme disease in mice. Prod. Natl. Acad. Sci. USA 94: 12533-12538

Special aspects of Lyme borreliosis and tick-borne encephalitis in the United States

9. Special aspects of Lyme borreliosis and tick-borne encephalitis in the United States

9.1. Introduction

The disease now known as Lyme borreliosis has a long and multinational history. In the United States, some aspects were recognized clinically long before the full scope of the disorder was appreciated. In the 1950's, general practitioners practicing in eastern Long Island, New York, an area highly endemic for Lyme disease, recognized an unusual form of recurrent, non-traumatic knee arthritis, referred to commonly as "Montauk knee". In retrospect these clearly were examples of Lyme arthritis.

In 1970, Rudy Scrimenti, an astute dermatologist practicing in Milwaukee, Wisconsin, recognized an unusual rash occurring in a hunter as being identical to erythema migrans, which had long been well described in the European literature. After consultation with several European colleagues, he treated this patient with antibiotics, with complete resolution of all symptoms.

The ensuing history is well known. In the mid 1970's, Steere investigated an apparent epidemic of juvenile rheumatoid arthritis in the area around Old Lyme, Connecticut, and in a series of detailed studies established the association of this disorder with tick bites, erythema migrans, and ultimately with the same constellation of neurologic disorders identified in European patients. This work culminated in the demonstration by the groups at Stony Brook and at Yale that this disorder was caused by a novel spirochete, which was named *Borrelia burgdorferi*, in honor of Willy Burgdorfer, it's original discoverer.

Prior to the identification of this disorder, tick borne disorders received relatively little attention in the American medical literature. Rocky Mountain Spotted Fever, caused by *Rickettsia rickettsii* a well known and potentially lethal disorder, is carried by the common dog tick, Dermatocenter variabilis in the eastern US, and D. andersoni in the west. In most cases this disease is easily treatable, particularly if identified early, and has not been the subject of much recent study. Tick bite paralysis, a toxin-mediated disorder associated with bites of several different species of ticks is unusual and has garnered little attention. The tick-borne encephalitis viruses, which cause a quite common problem in Europe and Asia, are fortunately quite rare in North America. Human infections with Powassan virus, the principle representative of this group of flaviviruses in the US, are extraordinarily rare.

Tick-borne diseases, particularly Lyme borreliosis, are quite geographically localized in North America. Lyme is quite prevalent in an enlarging swath along the eastern seaboard, now extending from New Hampshire to Delaware. A second endemic focus occurs in the upper Midwest, in a fairly localized region of Minnesota and Wisconsin (where Dr. Scrimenti's first case became infected). A third focus occurs in northern California. Although scattered cases have been reported elsewhere, these three areas account for the overwhelming majority of American Lyme disease. All locations are dictated by the coincidental occurrence of *Ixodes* ticks, a reservoir of infected hosts (typically field mice), a supporting population of deer or bears which facilitate maturation of the ticks, and coincidental and inadvertent invasion of humans into this ecosystem.

9.2. Characteristics of the pathogen

The properties of *Borrelia burgdorferi*, the pathogen responsible for Lyme borreliosis, are well described in the accompanying section. The principle difference is the far greater genetic homogeneity of American strains. Virtually all North American cases are caused by *B. burgdorferi sensu stricto*. This homogeneity presumably reflects a common origin of North American strains, thought to be related to the introduction of the disease with a single herd of deer to the Long Island/ Connecticut region early in the 20th century.

This homogeneity creates two significant advantages for American clinicians. First, the greater antigenic similarity among pathogenic strains simplifies immunodiagnosis - single immunoassays recognize virtually all strains. Second, immunization is more practical. Both vaccines that have been studied extensively have employed recombinant Outer Surface Protein A (OspA). The fact that these proteins are quite similar among all infecting strains makes a fairly simple vaccine practical. The same vaccine may well be less protective in European populations, because of the greater strain diversity.

Fortunately Powassan virus, the only tick-borne flavivirus that occurs in North America, while generally typical of all flaviviruses, rarely causes human disease.

9.3. Tick ecology and epidemiology

In North America the principle hard shelled tick vector for *B. burgdorferi* is *Ixodes scapularis* (initially erroneously thought to represent a novel species, named *Ixodes dammini*); in California *Ixodes pacificus* appears to be the principle vector. *Ixodes scapularis* occurs in temperate, low lying, damp environments, such as along the eastern seaboard of the United States and in the upper Midwest, such as Minnesota and Wisconsin, a region with myriad small lakes, ultimately feeding into the Mississippi and several other major North American rivers. These regions support the major hosts for these ticks - small mammals such as white footed and other mice, so important for the immature tick forms, and large mammals such as deer (on the east coast) or bears (in the Midwest), the hosts preferred by the adults for their final meals and mating.

The tick life cycle is thought to typically span two years, from the egg hatching into a larval form, having its initial blood meal, maturing into a nymphal form, partaking of a second blood meal, over-wintering and maturing into an adult, then again eating, mating, laying its eggs, and dying. Since transovarial transmission of spirochetes occurs rarely, maintenance of an endemic focus requires a reservoir of infected and relatively asymptomatic hosts, such as field mice or other small animals. The terminal meal and mating require the presence of the large host, such as deer or bears. Endemic foci have been maintained in the absence of these large hosts, presumably as ticks have selected secondary targets of opportunity, such as raccoons; however deer exclosure has been shown to decrease the incidence of infection significantly.

In California, with its more temperate climate, the life cycle is slightly different. I. pacificus, the tick responsible for transmission, feeds on lizards, which are far less likely to have the prolonged spirochetemia that is needed to permit ready infection of ticks. Moreover, these ticks may go through their entire life cycle in a single year, since the warmer climate makes over-wintering unnecessary.

9.4. Pathogenesis

The host immune response, and disease pathogenesis, are obviously identical regardless of whether the infection occurs in Europe, Asia or North America. However, there are some differences in clinical manifestations in these different locales, presumably reflecting subtle differences in tissue tropisms of the *Borrelia* strains that are locally prevalent. Although rheumatologic symptoms occur in European patients, they appear to be more frequent in the US. This probably is more than a bias of ascertainment in the clinicians treating these patients. Factors that might contribute to this difference include strain differences in the offending *Borrelia*, differences in prior human experience of the host, co-infection with other tick-borne pathogens, or differences in the genetically determined immune responses of the host. Of these potential differences, available data only supports the first - there are known strain differences between European and North American *Borrelia*. Although other factors might contribute, to date none has been shown to be significant.

9.5. Clinical Symptoms

Organ involvement in Lyme borreliosis tends to follow a temporal sequence, although the division into three distinct stages is probably somewhat arbitrary, and not clearly of clinical benefit. As in any infection, it is reasonable to conceptualize disease as acute and localized (analogous to stage I), acute and disseminated (similar to stage II) and late disseminated. At what point the syndrome becomes "late" is somewhat arbitrary; it is probably more useful to separate syndromes on the basis of degree of resultant end organ damage, rather than invoke a time limit.

In prospective American studies of children, a subpopulation that is much more closely observed than adults, as many as 90 % of those who develop Lyme borreliosis develop erythema migrans. As indicated above, in American series, dissemination with multiple erythema migrans appears to be more common than in Europe. As in Europe, the Centers for Disease Control recommended in 1990 that, for epidemiologic definition, an erythema migrans should be defined as an expanding erythema, at least 5 cm in diameter, lasting for days to weeks, and evolving over time. In most circumstances this will satisfactorily differentiate this cutaneous lesion from other erythroderms, tinea and other skin lesions.

Although it is often stated that nervous system involvement is more common in European populations, the only prospective studies that have addressed this issue have indicated that approximately 15 % of infected patients develop neurologic abnormalities, the same incidence as cited above in European patients. Informal comparisons of the incidence of the most severe form of involvement, encephalomyelitis, indicate a comparable incidence of about 0.5 cases/ year/100,000 population at risk in Austria, Scandinavia, and the northeast United States.

Joint involvement does appear to be more common in the United States. This tends to be a relapsing, large joint, asymmetric oligoarthritis, with particularly frequent involvement of knees, elbows and other large joints. Joints tend to be involved one at a time, with painful swelling, occurring and subsiding spontaneously. Although antibiotic therapy can end this syndrome, some individuals, particularly those with HLA DR3 and DR4 tend to develop persistent joint symptoms and destruction, and may require additional therapy.

Among cutaneous abnormalities, lymphadenosis cutis benigna occurs rarely. Acrodermatitis appears to be extraordinarily rare in North America, presumably reflecting unique properties of *B. afzelii*.

Nervous system involvement is quite comparable to that seen in Europe. During subacute dissemination, lymphocytic meningitis is quite common. At the same time patients may develop involvement of the cranial nerves, particularly the facial nerve, resulting in facial paralysis, which may be bilateral. Other cranial nerves may be involved less commonly, resulting in diplopia, facial pain or vertigo. Lower cranial nerves are involved less commonly - a pattern typical of cranial nerve involvement in basilar meningitides. Peripheral nerve involvement is commonplace; clinically this most commonly presents as a painful mono- or oligoradicular picture with sciatica-like pain, often with corresponding segmental weakness. When severe, there is often involvement of the spinal cord at the same level, with myelopathic signs and symptoms. In most instances peripheral nerve involvement can be demonstrated to be due to a mononeuropathy multiplex, suggesting a vasculopathic mechanism. The clinical presentation can be highly varied, depending on location and intensity - some patients develop a mild diffuse neuropathic picture, some a painful plexopathy, and others, the focal radicular picture.

In rare patients there is direct involvement of the brain and spinal cord. This most commonly presents as a myelopathic picture but can have hemispheral signs as well, with alterations of consciousness and focal abnormalities. This can respond to antimicrobial therapy, although some neurologic residua can occur, if inflammation has caused significant tissue destruction.

Although instances of apparent CNS vasculitis have been attributed to Lyme borreliosis, this remains less than clear-cut. While vasculitis is commonplace with late CNS syphilis, this seems to be at best rare with Lyme borreliosis and it is probably best to reserve judgement when patients with strokes are thought to have Lyme borreliosis as the cause.

The disorder that has given rise to the most diagnostic controversy has been the confusional state, or encephalopathy - a concept that has been much discussed, and frequently misunderstood. There are probably at least three settings in which patients with Lyme borreliosis develop alterations of cognitive function. By far the most common is the state seen in patients with disseminated infection, systemic symptoms and mildly impaired cognition and memory. This state is entirely analogous to the "toxic-metabolic" encephalopathy seen frequently in patients with other systemic inflammatory or infectious processes, is entirely reversible, and is not indicative of nervous system infection. This probably reflects the effect of cytokines, or related molecules, on the nervous system. Because it is not caused by CNS infection, cerebrospinal fluid, brain MRI scans and neurologic assessments are normal.

The second, and less common disorder, may be somewhat more severe, and probably reflects a mild form of the previously mentioned encephalomyelitis. These patients typically have CSF abnormalities - a pleocytosis, elevated CSF protein, and/or intrathecal production of anti-*Borrelia* antibodies; brain MRI's commonly demonstrate small areas of increased signal.

The third, which has been described in patients both in the United States and Europe, occurs in some patients after what is normally curative antibiotic treatment. This has been referred to as post-Lyme syndrome. Its pathogenesis is unresolved at this time. In some individuals, it may represent persistent infection. In others it may be due to persistent immune activation impacting on CNS function. In others it may indicate that the initial diagnosis of Lyme borreliosis was inaccurate. Each instance must be assessed individually.

Although numerous case reports suggest an extraordinary additional panoply of syndromes associated with this infection, a careful reading of the systematic literature indicates that Lyme borreliosis actually causes a distinct spectrum of disorders. Although it is always possible that further study will reveal additional syndromes linked to this infection, the fact that this disorder has been well known in Europe for over 8 decades, and in the United States for almost 3, makes it unlikely that additional disorders are commonly caused by it.

9.6. Diagnostics

Diagnosis of Lyme borreliosis in any given individual is dependent on three different elements - plausible epidemiologic exposure, a clinical syndrome within the defined spectrum associated with this infection, and laboratory support for the diagnosis. Although in any given patient one of these elements may be absent, without at least two the diagnosis must be considered only with the greatest circumspection.

This infection occurs in geographically well defined areas. In heavily urbanized areas, or regions remote from the previously described endemic foci, infection is virtually impossible to acquire. The clinical syndromes have been well described in the previous chapters. In endemic areas, there will be individuals with serologic evidence of exposure to this organism, who will develop other disorders - such as fractured legs, appendicitis, psychoses, etc. Obviously the presence of a positive test in a potentially exposed individual cannot be automatically assumed to prove causation of an atypical clinical disorder.

Laboratory support for the diagnosis rests largely on serologic testing. With the exception of the cutaneous manifestations, the bacterial burden is rather low. Since the spirochete requires special culture medium that is not widely available, and since it's doubling time in vitro is quite slow, diagnosis by culture, starting with a sample containing only a small number of organisms, is painfully difficult. Polymerase chain reaction testing, which can detect single genomic copies of the organism, has been quite disappointing, both due to problems with contamination, and to difficulties with sampling. It is entire possible that in 2 typical aliquots of spinal fluid from one patient, one may contain an organism while another may not. Other techniques, including measurement of immune complexes, immunofluorescent amplification of blood cultures, urine antigen testing and others, remain incompletely substantiated in the peer reviewed literature and remain subjects for future research, but not reliable means for clinical diagnosis.

Serologic testing, primarily using ELISA technology, remains the mainstay of laboratory testing. It is essential to realize that early in infection, such as at the time of the erythema migrans, many individuals will not yet have developed a sufficiently prominent antibody response to permit sero-diagnosis. In the presence of a typical rash, this should in no way impede the diagnosis. Similarly in rare circumstances, patients may never develop a positive antibody response. In general this has occurred in individuals who received inadvertent and non-curative doses of antibiotics very early in the course of infection, abrogating the normal maturation of the immune response.

In central nervous system infection diagnosis is greatly aided by examining spinal fluid. In the vast majority of patients with CNS - but not necessarily those with peripheral nervous system - infection spinal fluid will be abnormal. This may be non-specific, such as finding elevated CSF protein, a pleocytosis, the presence of oligoclonal bands or a relative increase in total intrathecal production of immunoglobulins, or more specific, with demonstrable production of specific anti-*B. burgdorferi* antibodies within the CNS. In the absence of CNS syphilis (which causes cross reactions in most anti-*Borrelia* assays) the latter finding is extremely compelling evidence of CNS infection. Its one limitation is that apparent antibody production may persist for years after curative treatment.

Serologic diagnosis has been greatly aided by the use of Western blots. This technique is most useful for differentiating weak false positive results from true positives. Unfortunately, this method is already being widely misinterpreted, in that "positive" blots in the face of negative ELISA's are being used to diagnose Lyme borreliosis. In general, in the presence of insufficient antibody to render an ELISA even weakly reactive, interpretation of a Western blot is extremely treacherous. Western blots are usually interpreted as negative or positive based on epidemiologically determined criteria. In individuals possessing 5 of the listed IgG bands, or 2 of the listed IgM bands, a diagnosis of exposure to this organism is quite secure (☞ Table 9.1). Unfortunately both criteria have significant false negative rates - approximately 68 % with the IgM criteria in early disease, and 17 % with the IgG criteria in more established infection. Therefore interpretation of negative Western blots requires some thoughtfulness.

IgG (5 of 10)	IgM (2 of 3)
18 kD	
23 kD	23 kD
28 kD	
30 kD	
39 kD	39 kD
41 kD	41 kD
45 kD	
60 kD	
66 kD	
93 kD	

Table 9.1: Western Blot Criteria

9.7. Therapy and Prognosis

In those individuals in whom the diagnosis of Lyme borreliosis is clear, treatment response is generally excellent. In early cutaneous disease treatment with doxycycline, amoxicillin or cefuroxime is highly effective. Treatment with agents such as azithromycin may be useful, but the response rate is probably less. Even in individuals with more advanced disease - meningitis, arthritis or other manifestations, oral agents may well be effective. However, it is commonplace to use parenteral regimens (ceftriaxone or cefotaxime) for nervous system involvement. The same regimens are used in those individuals who respond incompletely to oral treatment.

Duration of therapy remains somewhat controversial. In early disease, 2 to 3 week courses are typically used. When parenteral medications are employed, the few studies that have been performed indicate that statistically 2 weeks is as effective as. However, all the major centers treating large numbers of these patients have observed occasional unequivocal relapses in some patients who received only 2 weeks of treatment. As a result, 4-week courses are routinely employed when using these agents.

Although clinically response is usually apparent, improvement can be delayed. Patients with Lyme arthritis may continue to have joint symptoms for months after completing successful treatment. Those rare patients with structural CNS damage may have persistent abnormalities on exam, and on imaging studies. Serologic tests revert to normal either slowly or not at all, particularly in the spinal fluid. Non-specific markers of CNS infection, such as CSF cell count and protein typically improve, but this too can be a slow process.

Ultimately no laboratory procedure can provide unequivocal proof of cure - hence the presence of great uncertainty in this field. However it can safely be stated that statistically, the overwhelming majority of individuals receiving these courses of treatment will achieve microbiologic cure.

9.8. Prophylactic measures

The best methods of prevention of tick-borne infection are first, avoidance of ticks and second, early recognition and removal. Since infection generally requires at least 24 hours of tick attachment and feeding, a thorough tick check at the end of a day of possible exposure, with removal of any attached ticks (using a narrow tipped forceps inserted between the tick and the skin) provides the best protection. Wearing light colored clothes, with as little exposed skin as possible, minimizes the ticks' opportunities for attachment, and facilitates "tick spotting". Spraying clothes with acaricides can be useful; extensive and repeated skin spraying with these agents is ill-advised, particularly in small children, whose large surface to volume ratio puts them at risk of significant absorption, with development of potentially neurotoxic levels.

There is no evidence to date that prophylactic treatment of tick bites with systemic antibiotics is advantageous. In fact, the few systematic studies that have addressed this have indicated that the incidence of adverse reactions to drugs was equal to the rate of occurrence of infection, and that infection was always clinically obvious and easily treated.

Theoretically the most promising method of prevention is the development of a vaccine. Two vaccines have now been thoroughly studies in humans, and one is commercially available. Both have been demonstrated to confer substantial immunity, as summarized in the accompanying chapter.

Both appear to be safe, with no more reported untoward effects in individuals receiving the vaccine than in those receiving placebo. Both work by a rather novel method. The vaccine consists of recombinant OspA protein. This molecule has rather interesting properties. Although expressed by the spirochete in the tick, once the spirochete is exposed to the higher temperature of mammalian blood, expression is suppressed. As a result, humans rarely produce antibodies to this protein, at least early in disease. Since one of the theoretical fears about vaccination is that some neurologic and rheumatologic manifestations of this disorder may be due to immune-mediated processes, triggered by antigenic similarities between tick and host epitopes, it was hoped that immunization against a non-expressed peptide would make such a cross reaction less likely. Moreover, the lack of a host response to this marker in natural infection would make it simpler to tell - on Western blot - whether immunoreactivity in a patient's blood was due to immunization or infection. Finally, the relative homogeneity of OspA proteins in American populations makes such vaccination more likely to be effective than it may be in Europe.

Because these proteins are not expressed in infected patients, the effect of the vaccine-induced antibodies is rather unusual. When the tick ingests its blood meal, it also ingests antibody, thus attacking the spirochete *within the tick*! This Trojan horse approach appears to adequately suppress the number of spirochetes in the tick and limit the risk of infection.

This approach does have certain limitations. The ability of host antibody to suppress spirochetes is concentration dependent, and concentration obviously decreases over time. Consequently revaccination will almost certainly be necessary. Other than the inconvenience of requiring frequent (perhaps annual?) revaccination, it is by no means clear what the effect of repeated vaccinations will be on patients. Finally, patients must remember that while vaccination may well protect them from *B. burgdorferi*, it will offer no protection from other tick-borne pathogens such as *Ehrlichia or Babesia*. Thus the same protective measures will remain essential to avoid contracting one of these other disorders.

References

Benach JL, Bosler EM, Hanrahan JP, et al. Spirochetes isolated from the blood of two patients with Lyme Disease.. NEJM 1983;308:740-742

Benke T, Gasse T, Hittmair-Delazer M, Schmutzhard E. Lyme encephalopathy: long-term neuropsychological deficits years after acute neuroborreliosis. Acta Neurol Scand 1995;91:353-7

Control CfD. Lyme Disease - Case Definition. MMWR 1990;39:20-21

Dattwyler RJ, Halperin JJ, Volkman DJ, Luft BJ. Treatment of late Lyme disease. Lancet 19881191-3.

Dattwyler RJ, Luft BJ, Maladorno D, et al. Treatment of late Lyme disease - a comparison of 2 weeks vs 4 weeks of ceftriaxone. VII International Congress on Lyme Borreliosis. San Francisco, Calif, 1996:186

Dennis DT, Meltzer MI. Antibiotic prophylaxis after tick bites.Lancet 1997;350:1191-2r

Dressler F, Whalen JA, Reinhardt BN, Steere AC. Western blotting in the serodiagnosis of Lyme disease. J Infect Dis 1993;167:392-400

Halperin JJ, Luft BJ, Anand AK, et al. Lyme neuroborreliosis: central nervous system manifestations. Neurology 1989;39:753-759

Halperin JJ, Pass HL, Anand AK, Luft BJ, Volkman DJ, Dattwyler RJ. Nervous system abnormalities in Lyme disease. Ann N Y Acad Sci 1988; 539:24-34

Halperin JJ, Heyes MP. Neuroactive kynurenines in Lyme borreliosis. Neurology 1992;42:43-50

Logigian EL, Kaplan RF, Steere AC. Chronic neurologic manifestations of Lyme disease. N Engl J Med 1990;323:1438-1444

Luft BJ, Dattwyler RJ, Johnson RC, et al. Azithromycin compared with amoxicillin in the treatment of erythema migrans. Ann Int Med 1996; 124:785-791

Magid D, Schwartz B, Craft J, Schwartz JS. Prevention of Lyme disease after tick bites. A cost-effectiveness analysis [see comments]. N Engl J Med 1992;327:534-41

Pachner AR, Steere AC. Neurological findings of Lyme disease. Yale J Biol Med 1984;57:481-3

Pediatric Lyme Disease Study Group, Gerber MA, Shapiro ED, Burke GS, Parcells VJ, Bell GL. Lyme disease in children in southeastern Connecticut. N Engl J Med 1996;335:1270-4

Scrimenti RJ. Erythema chronicum migrans. Arch Dermatol 1970;102:104-105

Steere AC, Grodzicki RL, Kornblatt AN, et al. The spirochetal etiology of Lyme Disease. NEJM 1983;308:733-740

Steere AC, Dwyer E, Winchester R. Association of Chronic Lyme Arthritis with HLA-DR4 and HLA-DR2 Alleles. N Engl J Med 1990;323:219-23

List of abbreviations

10. List of abbreviations

Abbreviation	Term
Ab	antibody
ACA	acrodermatitis chronica atrophicans
AI	antibody index
ATP	adenosine triphosphate
ATR	Achilles tendon reflex
Bmp	**b**asic **m**embrane **p**rotein
BR	biceps reflex
BSK	Barbour-Stoenner-Kelly medium
C5a	fragment of fifth complement component (anaphylatoxin)
C3b	fragment of third complement component
C5b-9	complex of complement components C5, C6, C7, C8, and C9
CFT	complement fixation test
CNS	central nervous system
CT	computerized tomography
DNA	deoxyribonucleic acid
dNTP	deoxyribonucleoside triphosphate
EAEP	early auditory evoked potential
E[C]M	erythema (chronicum) migrans
EEG	electroencephalogram
ELISA	enzyme-linked immunosorbent assay
Epp	**ex**ported **p**rotein
HIT	hemagglutination-inhibition test
HSP	**h**eat **s**hock **p**rotein
ICAM-1	intercellular adhesion molecule-1
IFT	immunofluorescence test
IHAT	indirect hemagglutination test
IL-12	interleukin-12
IL-4	interleukin-4
IL-8	interleukin-8
IL-1β	interleukin-1β
INF-γ	interferon-γ
kb	kilobases
kD	kilodalton
LCB	lymphadenosis cutis benigna
MCP-1	monocyte chemoattractant protein-1
MIC	minimal inhibitory concentration
MRT	magnetic resonance tomography
NB	neuroborreliosis
NCR	non-coding region
NHS	normal human serum
NS	nonstructural protein of the TBE virus
NT	neutralization test
ORF	**o**pen **r**eading **f**rame
Osp	**o**uter **s**urface **p**rotein
p	protein
PAGE	polyacrylamide gel electrophoresis
PCR	polymerase chain reaction
PFGE	pulsed-field gel electrophoresis
PVDF	polyvinyl difluoride
RFLP	restriction fragment length polymorphism
RR	radial reflex
rRNA	ribosomal ribonucleic acid
RTBEV	Russian tick-borne encephalitis virus
RT	reverse transcriptase
RT-PCR	reverse transcriptase polymerase chain reaction
SDS	sodium dodecylsulfate (anionic detergent)
s.l.	sensu lato
SPECT	single photon emission computed tomography
s.s.	sensu stricto
TBE	tick-borne encephalitis
TH1	CD4-T-lymphocytes
TH2	CD4-T-lymphocytes
TNF-α	tumor necrosis factor α
VCAM-1	vascular adhesion molecule 1
VEP	visual evoked potential

Table 9.1: Summary of the abbreviations used in the text

Index

A

Acrodermatitis chronica atrophicans
    atrophic final stage 55
    case history 57
    description 56
    differential diagnosis 56
    discovery 16
    findings 55, 56
    inflammatory edematous phase 55
Afzelius, Artvid 16
Albumin ratio 83
Antibiotics against B. burgdorferi 88, 112
    CSF penetration 112
    MIC 88
Antibiotic sensitivity testing 87
Antibiotics, minimal inhibitory concentration of antibiotics .87
Antigen structure of B. burgdorferi 24
Antibody detection 91, 94, 107
    in the cerebrospinal fluid in neuroborreliosis 100
    in the cerebrospinal fluid in TBE 107

B

Bannwarth's syndrome 53, 59
Barbour, Alan 20
Barbour-Stoenner-Kelly medium 22, 86
Basal body 22
Basic membrane protein 24
Blebs 22, 45
Blood-brain barrier 83
BmpA 24
Borrelia
    afzelii 32
    andersonii 20
    burgdorferi 17, 20
    burgdorferi (sensu lato) 20, 32
    burgdorferi (sensu stricto) 32
    culture conditions 22
    culturing 87
    duttoni 20
    garinii 32
    genus 20
    group DN127 20
    hermsii 20
    japonica 20
    longitudinal section 21
    lusitaniae 20
    main protein components 24
    molecular biology aspects 22
    morphology 21
    persistence of 46
    recurrentis 20
    transverse section 21, 22
    valaisiana 20
Borrelia burgdorferi complex
    area of distribution 20
    classification 20
    pathogenicity 20
Borrelia burgdorferi infection 17

Borrelia chromosome 22
Borrelia infection
    disseminated 42
    local 42
    persistent 42
    stage I 42
    stage II 42
    stage III 42
Borrelia serology 92
    false negative 102
    false positive 102
    possible sources of error in diagnostics 102
    positive 99
    problems in the interpretation of findings 99
Borrelia-specific antigens, detection of 90
Borrelia strains, ultrasonicate extracts 25
BSK medium 22
Burgdorfer, Willy 16, 20

C

California encephalitis 34
Central European encephalitis 16, 25
Chorioretinitis 57, 71
Chromosome, linear 22
Complement-fixation reaction 93
Complement system 43
Complete-antigen immunoblot 95
Cross reactions 102
CSF analysis 83
    findings in neuroborreliosis 83
CSF penetration of antibiotics 112
CSF-serum antibody index 100

D

Dark-field microscopy 21
Dengue fever 34
Dermatoborreliosis 17, 54
Dissemination 43
DNA-DNA hybridization 20
Domains
    A 26
    B 26
    C 26

E

Eastern equine encephalitis 34
Electron microscopy 106
ELISA 107
    in borreliosis diagnostics 94
Encephalomyelitis 66
    case history 66
    clinical symptoms 66
    differential diagnosis 66
    progressive 60, 66
Endoflagella 21
    number 22
    structure 22
Envelope protein 26

EppA 24
Erythema migrans 54
  description 55
  differential diagnosis 55
  discovery 16
  findings 54, 55
  histopathology 55
  monitoring of treatment 115
  prognosis 115
  serology 99
Erythema migrans borreliosis 17
Exported protein A 24

F

Fasciitis 67
Flagellar filament 22
Flagellar hook 22
Flagellin 24
Flagellin (p41) 24

G

Garin-Bujadoux-Bannwarth syndrome 59
Gemmae 22
Gene sequence of the Borrelia chromosome 22
Germinal center macrophages 56
Glycoprotein prM/M 26

H

Haller's organ 32
Hard-bodied ticks 30
Hemagglutination test, indirect 93

I

Immune defense 45
  in TBE 49
Immunoblot, recombinant 96
Immunoblot technique 94
Immunofluorescence test, indirect 93
Immunopathology 47
Inoculation against TBE 38
Ixodes
  dammini 16
  reduvii 16
Ixodes ricinus
  antagonists 32
  body length 31
  developmental stages 31
  growth 32
  hosts 32, 33
  life cycle 30
  lifespan 31
  mouthparts 31
  occurrence 30

J

Japanese encephalitis 34

L

Lichen sclerosis et atrophicus 57
Lyme arthritis 16, 69
  changes in laboratory parameters 70
  characteristics of stage II/III 80
  chronic form 69

clinical symptoms 69
  differential diagnosis 70
  monitoring of treatment 117
  prognosis 117
  radiological findings 70
  serology 99
  stage II 117
  stage III 117
  synovial biopsy 70
Lyme borreliosis 20, 32
  acute organ manifestations 44
  assessment of therapeutic outcome 114
  cardinal symptoms 80
  chronic 34
  chronic organ manifestations 44
  course of infection 52
  delayed cure 118
  detection of antibodies 91
  detection of the pathogen by culture 86
  diagnostics 80
  direct pathogen detection 86
  discovery 16
  epidemiological data for selected countries 34
  immune defense 45
  immunization 125
  indirect pathogen detection 85
  inflammatory reaction 43
  instrumental examinations 80
  internistic manifestations 69
  local infection 42
  microbiological diagnostics 85
  microscopic pathogen detection 86
  monitoring of treatment 116
  NSAIDs 114
  number of new cases per year 32
  organ manifestations 54
  pathogen 32
  pathogenesis 42
  prognosis 118
  reactions after infection 43
  relapse 118
  stage dependence of the antibody pattern 92
  stages 52
  stage I 53
  stage II 53
  stage III 53
  standard serological diagnostics 97
  steroids 114
  syndromes 52
  taxonomic classification 20
  therapy 112, 113
  therapy during pregnancy 115
  therapy of stage I 113
  therapy of stage II 114
  therapy of stage III 115
  treatment resistance 118
  vaccine development 126
Lyme carditis 70
  characteristics of stage II 80
  histology 70
  symptoms 70
Lyme disease 17

Lyme encephalopathy 67
Lymphadenosis cutis benigna 55
    description 56
    differential diagnosis 56
    discovery 16
    findings 55
    histology 56

M

Membrane, trilaminar 21
Membrane proteins 25
Meningitis 62
    case history 62, 73
    clinical symptoms 62, 73
    differential diagnosis 73
    in TBE 73
Meningoencephal(oradicul)itis 62
    clinical symptoms 62
Meningoencephalitis 62, 74
    case history 63, 74, 75
    clinical symptoms 62, 74
    differential diagnosis 74
Meningomyel(oradicul)itis 61
    clinical symptoms 61
    differential diagnosis 62
Meningomyelitis 61
Meningoradiculitis
    case history 61
    cranial 60
    differential diagnosis 60
    lymphocytic 53
    serology 102
    spinalis 59
    spinalis et cranialis 60
Mono(poly)neuritis 57
Murray Valley encephalitis 34
Myelitis
    clinical symptoms 75
    differential diagnosis 76
Myeloradiculitis 57
Myositis 57, 67

N

Neuritis
    acute 67
    chronic 67
Neuroborreliosis 57
    age and sex distribution 58
    case history 65
    cerebrovascular 64
    changes in laboratory parameters 83
    characteristics of stage II/III 80
    detection of antibody synthesis 100
    diagnostic criteria 81
    findings 58
    frequency 57
    frequency of pathological findings 82
    histological findings 66
    monitoring of treatment 116
    MRT findings 65
    neurophysiological findings 63
    prognosis 116
    stage II 116
    symptoms 58
    syndromes 54, 59
New infections 46
Nonstructural protein 26

O

Old Lyme 16
Oms 24
Ophthalmoborreliosis 70
    case history 71
    clinical symptoms 71
Osp 24
    A 24
    B 24
    C 24
    D 24
    E 24
    F 24
OspA/OspC serotypes 21
OspA/OspC serotyping system 21
Outer surface protein 24, 45

P

p18 24
p83/100 24
"Paralysie par les tiques" 16
Paraplegic myelitis 57
Phase-contrast microscopy 21
Plasmids 22, 23
    circular 22
    gene sequence 22
    linear 22
    of various strains of Borrelia 23
Polymerase chain reaction
    principle 88
    value 89
Preimmune phase 45
Properties of the pathogen 20
Protein E 26
Protein bands 24
Protoplasm cylinder 21
Pulse therapy 118

Q

Quotient diagram, Reiber 102

R

Radiculitis
    clinical symptoms 75
    differential diagnosis 76
RFLP analysis 20
Relapsing fever 20
RT-PCR 105
Russian tick born encephalitis 16, 25

S

Scleroderma, circumscribed 57
SDS-PAGE 24
Serum bactericidal activity test 96
Simultaneous immunization 130
S layer 21
Soft-bodied ticks 30

Solid-phase IgM ELISA 94
Space, periplasmic 21
Species, differentiation of 91
Standardization of tests 102
St. Louis encephalitis 34
Synovial fluid 84

T

TBE
    antibody kinetics 106
    changes in laboratory parameters 103
    course of the disease 71
    diagnostics 104
    disease stages 72
    endemic regions 35, 36
    immunization 39
    immunoglobulins 119
    incidence 38
    instrumental examinations 103
    interpretation of findings 107
    magnetic resonance tomographic finding 104
    manifestations outside the nervous system 76
    manifestation phase 73
    mortality 37, 120
    occurrence 16
    organ manifestations and syndromes 73
    pathogen 34
    pathogenesis 47
    pathological findings 105
    possible course 48
    principal symptoms 104
    prodromal phase 72
    prognosis 119
    reactions after infection 48
    regions with an increased risk of infection 36
    risk of infection as a result of tick bites 37
    therapy 119
    vaccine complications 128
    vaccine side effects 128
    vaccination 127
TBE-prophylaxis
    fast immunization 127
    long-term regimen 127
TBE virus
    antigen structure 26
    detection of antibodies 105
    direct detection techniques 106
    genetic organization 26
    genus 25
    indirect detection techniques 105
    molecular biology aspects 26
    related flaviviruses 25
    schematic diagram 26
    structure 25
    subtype 1 25
    subtype 2 25
    taxonomic classification 25
Tick control 125
Tick-borne encephalitis 16
Tick borreliosis 17
Tick ecology 30

Ticks
    classification 30
    general protection measures 124
    general introduction 30
    geographic distribution 33
    infection levels 33
    pathogenic microorganisms 30
    removal 124
    risk of infection 37
Typing procedures for B. burgdorferi 91

V

Vaccination against SSE 127
Vascular reactions in the area of inflammation 43
Venezuelan equine encephalitis 34
Vesicle types in borrelias 22
Virus culture 105
Virus detection 105

W

West Nile encephalitis 34
Western equine encephalitis 34
Western blot technique 94
'Wood tick' 30

Y

Yellow fever 34